Learning Lessons

Learning Lessons

Medicine, Economics, and Public Policy

Rashi Fein

Transaction Publishers
New Brunswick (U.S.A.) and London (U.K.)

Library of Congress Catalog Number: 2009044444
ISBN: 978-1-4128-1080-7
Printed in the United States of America

Library of Congress Cataloging-in-Publication Data

Fein, Rashi.
    Learning lessons : medicine, economics, and public policy / Rashi Fein.
        p. ; cm.
    Includes bibliographical references and index.
    ISBN 978-1-4128-1080-7 (alk. paper)
        1. Medical policy. 2. Medical economics. I. Title.
    [DNLM: 1. Health Policy--economics--United States. 2. Cost-Benefit Analysis--United States. 3. Public Policy--economics--United States. 4. Social Responsibility--United States. 5. Social Values--United States. WA 540 AA1 F299L 2010]

RA393.F45 2010
338.4'73621--dc22

                                                        2009044444

For Family, Friends, Colleagues, and Students
Who Encouraged This Project

Contents

Acknowledgments

It is impossible to name all those to whom I am indebted for their contributions to this book. The lessons I have learned, the matters that interest me, the priorities I set, and the values I hold – thus, the discussion in the material that follows – have been influenced by the books I have read, the songs I have heard, the conversations I have had, and above all by the people with whom I have intersected on a face to face basis or by reading or hearing about them. Even were I able to construct such a list, it would be far too long to be included.

Nevertheless, there are some to whom I am especially indebted, individuals without whose influence you, the reader, would not be able to hold this volume in your hands. Certainly that list includes all who are mentioned in the various stories and lessons in the pages that follow. It also includes family and friends on whom I practiced "story telling" as well as former students who heard a number of these lessons in class and, in that sense "vetted" the material. Even more directly involved were the Robert Wood Johnson Foundation Scholars in Health Policy and their faculties at the University of California (Berkeley), University of Michigan, Yale University, and Harvard University. Once a year, in a period stretching over a decade, I had an opportunity to open the annual research conference that the Foundation sponsored for program participants. It was in those remarks that I shared some of the lessons I had learned and the stories behind them. The way my comments were received encouraged me to believe there might be some value in sharing these matters with a larger audience.

Even so it is not clear that I would have done the work required to think seriously about the things that I have learned over my professional career, to organize them around themes, and to create a manuscript. To undertake all that – to produce something so different from the other books I've written which were research based and exclusively in the health field – required periodic encouragement. I benefitted from continuing expressions of interest, my own awareness that books do not write themselves, and the frequent inquiry: "how is the book coming?" I owe the greatest debt to three colleagues who were and remain deeply involved in the Scholars' program, who are vitally interested in public policy, and who kept telling me that "there's a book there:" Alan Cohen of Boston University, James Morone of Brown University, and Mark Peterson of the University of California (Los Angeles).

That threesome provided the mixture of encouragement and goading and, importantly, helped convince me that some anecdotes I shared with them simply because I found them interesting belonged in the book. They all read the manuscript and offered their valuable comments. Their perspective served as a reminder that persons from other disciplines and with different backgrounds might derive different lessons from the events recounted and, therefore, that I should attempt to write for a broader audience. Five people know how important Cohen, Morone, and Peterson were to this project: those three, my wife, and I.

I also want to acknowledge and especially single out the contribution made by three other individuals who read parts or all of the manuscript and who offered numerous helpful comments: my sister-in-law, Bernice Breslau; my brother, Leonard Fein; and my good friend and sometime collaborator, Julius B. Richmond.

A very special thank you is due Ms. Jacqueline Wehmueller, executive editor, The Johns Hopkins University Press. I deeply appreciate her interest and the hours she spent reading and discussing various drafts. Her comments were both instructive and invaluable.

I also want to thank Transaction Publishers and its talented staff members. I especially single out Irving Louis Horowitz who, because of his breadth of vision in and about the social sciences, believed in the manuscript's potential. No manuscript becomes a book without passing through the hands of an editor. I was fortunate to encounter Larry Mintz to whom I and the readers owe a debt of gratitude.

Introduction

A story my father used to tell:

When I was a little boy of nine in a far away city called Bendery, in a far away country called Rumania, my teacher, Reb Haimke was teaching us Leviticus and said: "Children, it is told that far, far away there is a land called America and I know that is so. It is also told that in that land there is a city named Philadelphia and I suppose that also is true. And I have heard that in that city called Philadelphia there is a huge bell and that on that bell are engraved the words from Leviticus, 'Proclaim liberty throughout all the land unto all the inhabitants thereof.' And they tell me that is the law of the land. Now, I really have a hard time believing *that*. Liberty for all the inhabitants of the land! Unbelievable! I can *imagine* such a proclamation, such a law, but I can't really *believe* it. Still, they say it is so. So, children, when you grow up you might go to America, maybe even to the city called Philadelphia. If you do, see whether all this is true and if it really is so, if there is such a bell and such a law, send some of America back to Bendery; we so badly need it.[1]

Continuing, my father would tell us that fifteen years later he and my mother left the University of Vienna where they were students and came to America and then, because of a family connection, to Philadelphia. There, in Independence Hall, they saw the bell and read the words from Leviticus on what we know as the Liberty Bell: "Proclaim liberty throughout all the land unto all the inhabitants thereof."

But then they noticed that the bell was cracked. And as time passed, as they became Americans, they realized that the crack, too, conveyed a message about America. It took almost one hundred years from the founding of the Republic for slavery to be abolished. And even then emancipation did not mean that liberty for all had yet been achieved. The 1920s, when my parents came here, were the days of the Ku Klux Klan and lynchings, of economic slavery and union busting, of the execution of Sacco and Vanzetti, of Red

1

scares, of the enactment of discriminatory immigration laws. It was a time in which racism and anti-Semitism flourished and signs "whites only" and "no Jews, blacks, or dogs allowed" were not uncommon.

That was how my father would explain why he and my mother became "bell-menders." They were determined to repair the crack, to make real the proclamation of liberty throughout all the land unto all the inhabitants thereof, to close the gap between where we were and where we could be, between the American reality and the American idea and ideal.

I have been concerned with public policy for almost as long as I can recall, undoubtedly because I grew up in a home of bell-menders, in a household that was deeply interested in public affairs. Domestic and international politics were the usual topics of conversation at our supper table. My parents believed that if "life was unfair"—as it often was—government was the instrument that could help make it fairer. They, along with millions of other Americans, were convinced that only government could bring the nation out of the depths of the Great Depression, that only government could mount effective opposition to Fascist and Nazi aggression, that government was a necessary institution.

I was raised in the atmosphere of 1930s liberal politics, with its emphasis on civil liberties, civil rights, and greater equity in the distribution of income and wealth. Government "of the people, by the people, for the people" was the instrument through which these concerns and commitments could be achieved. It was government that administered the progressive tax system, provided free public education and libraries, owned and operated hospitals and transportation systems, built roads and harbors, regulated the prices that monopolies such as water, electricity, and telephone charged. It was through the collective action of government, an instrument of social solidarity, that one could build a better world.

Furthermore, my parents and I—as many others—believed in a most activist role for the federal government in contrast with what was expected from states and local jurisdictions. In no small measure this was because at the time that I was growing up and for many years both before and after, there was a healthy skepticism—to use a mild term—about the progress that states, let alone cities, could make in achieving the necessary redistribution of income and of wealth. This did not simply reflect the vast taxing and spending power of the federal government, a power that states and municipalities lacked. It was also because many states were led by openly racist power structures, including governors, legislators, and judges who did not and would not provide equal opportunity and greater equity to all their citizens, most especially those of color. The white leadership in those states may have articulated a policy of "separate and equal," but truly believed in policies that in largest measure were calculated to be "separate and unequal." In contrast, though the federal government was certainly not devoid of racism, there were offsets to the power of legislators who represented pro-segregation states. Less monolithic, the federal government offered hope.

The belief in government and in the role that government could play was coupled with—indeed, dependent on—a strong belief in American democracy and in liberty and justice. Quite often my father reminded me that his admiration for America was strong, indeed perhaps stronger than mine. After all, he had chosen America while I was here because of an accident of birth. The story of the Liberty Bell may or may not have been based on fact, but in its deepest sense it was true.

That is why every spring, with all the family and many friends at the Passover Seder table celebrating the Festival of Freedom, he would tell the Liberty Bell story. In time it became the connecting tissue of my political consciousness. Indeed, in time I have taken up the tradition and the guests at my Seder table hear it every year

Perhaps it was that story enjoining me to help mend the bell that helped broaden what otherwise might have been a limited "academic" interest in history and public policy. Doubtless there were other stories as well, all pointing in the same direction. Surely they were with me when I served in the United States Navy during World War II. Later they fueled my desire to participate in what John F. Kennedy pledged would be "an Administration that will get this country moving again" bringing me to Washington and to a position on the staff of the President's Council of Economic Advisers

(CEA) in the early months of the Kennedy administration.

That a person with a policy bent would be drawn to Washington and to the new and young administration in 1961 is not at all surprising. I and many other economists had been educated by mentors who had told us about the hard work, excitement, and, above all, sense of accomplishment they had experienced when they had worked for the federal government during the New Deal and/or during the Second World War. They felt, indeed they knew, that they had made a difference. In 1961, we wanted to believe—we did believe—that the Kennedy administration represented our opportunity to be part of what we felt would be the great adventure of our time. We took the idea of a "New Frontier" quite seriously and were deeply moved by JFK's inaugural address. What I and my colleagues could do seemed clear: help repair the Liberty Bell.

Nevertheless, in spite of Washington's attractions, it would be a mistake to suppose that an interest in public policy must necessarily lead to the nation's capital. "Policy" is not a word that applies solely to public policy decisions made in Washington and "policy maker" and "policy adviser" are not terms reserved solely for powerful elected or appointed members of the various branches of the federal government and to those who work with and for them. Nor would it be sufficient to expand the definition to include all those with similar responsibilities in state and local government. The word "policy" and the phrase "makes policy" also apply to actions and individuals outside of government.

Policy is not only about what takes place in Washington, in the state house, in the courthouse, or in town hall. My dictionary defines "policy" quite broadly: "a principle, plan or course of action, as pursued by a government, organization, individual, etc." Policy decisions involve the selection of this path or that, the choice made between or among alternatives, the judgment to pursue this goal and shelve some other. Policy, therefore, is an everyday event and policy development takes place in all kinds of settings. True, some policies regarding war or peace, approval or rejection of a new drug or therapeutic intervention, altering the federal tax code, raising highway tolls, or extending the school day, are made by government officials and legislators and affect millions of persons.

But "policy" also includes decisions made in the private sector: expanding the emergency room in the community hospital, moving the local shirt factory abroad, offering health benefits to part-time employees, being indifferent to discrimination against women. Those, too, are policy choices—as are the choices made by families and individuals when they select among alternative courses of action: saving or spending, buying a house or renting, having one's children attend public or private school, watching TV or joining a choral group.

Of course, few of us think of ourselves as policy makers. Furthermore, we are not at all certain that we consider folks who are extremely interested in and who live and breathe "policy" as appropriate "role models." Indeed, we sometimes use the term "policy wonk" as a pejorative; some, perhaps many, parents may not want their offspring to grow up to be or marry one. While many of us know what we want—better schools, a reformed health care financing and delivery system, a healthier housing market, lower taxes, smaller deficits—we cannot easily choose among the different policies we are told are required to attain our goals. We are likely to be more interested and knowledgeable about the broad picture than about the details of the legislation, proposed regulations, or court decisions, all of which "make policy" by taking account of the nuances of words.

We think of policy as something that belongs to "them" and not to us. We aren't senators, mayors, city councilors, members of the zoning council, or hospital directors. When it comes to policy we think of ourselves as "little people." Nevertheless, we are not only affected by policies made by others, we do make policy. Paraphrasing Moliere's comment about prose, each of us could write: "Good heavens! For more than forty years I have been making policy without knowing it."[2] Still—for reasons that are clear—private individual and family decisions are not the subject of my inquiry.

Policy choices do not burst forth full blown in some explosion of insight. They emerge as part of a process in which choices are debated, developed, altered, amended, modified, refined, and taken "back to the drawing board" for change. In government and large private organizations, most often that process, involving task forces, committees, commissions, or working groups, does not include the "principals" who will make the final decisions and exercise the ultimate choices, those whose names we know and whose power we acknowledge. Yet, those who are the staff members and the assistants, those who create the menu of choices that are placed before the "decision makers" are a vital part of the policy process. Often they are anonymous individuals. But it is they who determine the available options and present the advantages and disadvantages of each.

As a staff member of the Council of Economic Advisers, I once was part of a group of policy analysts who were asked to prepare a range of choices for our "principals," all high officials in the executive branch of the Kennedy administration. The then director of the Bureau of the Budget (the precursor to today's Office of Management and Budget) met with us to set forth the context for our deliberations. He made it clear that he wanted our report to present as wide a range of choices as possible and as thorough an analysis as feasible. He told us, "I can discard something you put in, but I can't add what you omitted." To ignore the contribution made and—within limits—the power exercised by agenda developers and advisers is to overlook a vital part of the policy process.

The restaurant diner makes the final choice from the menu put before her, but it is the chef who determines the range of choice. The patron who was offered only halibut, haddock, or flounder cannot select sea bass. Yet, if time after time the menu is too sparse and the choices appear too limited, she may decide to choose a different chef and restaurant. The same holds for the "decision maker" who needs to be wise enough to know when too much has been left unsaid and who, if that is the case, may select a different set of advisers. In that sense, of course, ultimate authority rests with the "principal," the official whose name we know. That, indeed, is where "the buck stops." Yet, the influence of staff on the policy options and decisions should not be underestimated.

This is a book about the policy process, the considerations that advisers have or should have in mind as they develop and select among alternatives, the ways that each of us might want to think about making decisions, and the lessons we should remember in order to minimize avoidable errors. In writing I will share stories of some of my experiences in government, the classroom, and private life. The anecdotes and situations I describe are not designed to present a rounded theory about public administration or a comprehensive treatment of important components of political science. Like most of us, I, as almost all the people with whom I worked on policy initiatives, came to that work from another discipline—in my case economics—without the formal training that one might receive today in a school of government or public policy. Perhaps the experience of "finding my own way" through action and experience rather than through theory will appear quaint. But perhaps the successes, the failures, and the lessons I learned, may illuminate the process and prove useful and at least occasionally inspirational.

Having confessed that I was educated as an economist, I should alert the reader that I will advance as a central thesis—a number of stories will illustrate that thesis—the proposition that an effective adviser must bring knowledge and interests that extend beyond the confines of a single discipline, even one as methodologically powerful as economics. Unless the adviser presents a range of choices developed with contributions from many field of knowledge, the proposed policies are likely to be far too constrained and, at worst, to be unworkable. As an economist perhaps I am especially sensitive to the need to expand one's vision beyond economics.

Nevertheless, the separate examination of economics is justified by the important role it plays in developing and assessing policy and in evaluating performance. Economics is a powerful discipline that has a pattern of analysis and thought conducive to examining choices, balancing the pros and cons and benefits and costs, and weighing alternative incentives to induce different behaviors. Economists are well-trained in statistical analysis and mathematical techniques that enable them to extract conclusions from bodies of data that often appear ambiguous or even impenetrable. These several attributes enable them to present findings that some principals may feel cannot easily be disputed—and therein lies a danger. While aware and respectful of the contribution that economic analysis can make to discussions of policy, I want to guard against a belief that by itself economics can provide "all the answers." Reliance on economics while ignoring the richer approach of political economy and the potential contributions of such subjects as history, sociology, psychology, and political science runs serious risks of incompleteness and consequent error. The limitations of pure economics, therefore, bear careful examination. On that matter the perspective this book takes is easily summarized: there is more to life and to our and our nation's welfare than economics. We live in a society, not in an economy.

In the first chapter, I elaborate on the role of economics and of economic criteria in developing and establishing policy. I raise issues involving the measurement and comparison of benefits and costs of various actions and I examine the degree to which one's policy recommendations should be shaped by an economic calculus as contrasted with a broader social perspective. As context for this discussion, I provide some biographical material on how I entered the field of economics, selected the area of interest within it, and came to respect what economists have to say about policy and at the same time increasingly to value the contribution that other disciplines can make.

Since policy development and policy debate necessarily involve discussion and communication, my second chapter addresses the meaning and influence of words, the components of the language through which policy is presented. Many years ago when I was a graduate student in political economy at the Johns Hopkins University a group of us appealed to our most senior professor, Fritz Machlup, asking that the department recognize mathematics as one of the "languages" meeting the traditional Ph.D. requirement that the candidate have a working knowledge of two foreign languages. We had heard that the University of Chicago had decided to accept mathematics as a "second" language and believed that precedent would strengthen our case and prove convincing. Our plea was rejected with the quite "radical" argument for the late 1940s that it was a given that every economist had to know mathematics. Therefore, it followed that if our suggestion were accepted, Ph.D. candidates would know math and one foreign language.

Conversely, under the existing rules we'd still know math and an additional two languages. Not surprisingly, we were told the latter was preferable.

Some few years later we came to realize that the real problem was that Machlup did not really believe that mathematics was a language. In a debate (at an annual meeting of the American Economic Association) on the use of mathematics in economics he disputed the view articulated by that great economist, Paul Samuelson, that one should not fear mathematics, that it was "just another language," but a powerful one with the advantage of absolute precision rather than the disadvantage of ambiguity. Hearing that, Machlup, drew himself up and with some scorn asked, "Simply a language like other languages? Can one really say in mathematics whatever one might say in English? If it is just a language [and now leaning forward and adopting a sultry tone that he had undoubtedly brought with him from Vienna] how do you say 'love' in mathematics?"

Though mathematics and statistics have become ever more important in economics over the ensuing years, policy discourse still takes place in a language that uses words. All of us who have wished we had employed some other words in trying to make a case for our point of view on this or that issue are painfully aware that the choice of words and their emotional overlay can make or break an argument. It, therefore, is no accident that a number of my stories will examine the power of words, their meaning, and their influence on policy formulation and development.

In the third chapter, I discuss one of the most basic issues that the policy adviser must address in developing policy alternatives: how wide to cast the policy net, how broad the menu of options. This question of scope takes many forms: the choice between what might be called "vision" and "political realism," the choice between answering the question asked because it was the question that was asked and concluding that it was the wrong question and that one's principals as well as principles will be better served by addressing the "correct" issue; the choice between opting for a marginal, more rapidly implemented change and a larger change with greater impact, but requiring more time for implementation and adjustment; the choice between incremental and comprehensive change. The various stories that illustrate those kinds of choices remind us that in a very real sense how decision makers and their advisers deal with the agenda and its timing are among the most basic policy decisions they make.

The fourth chapter reminds us that since policy is developed by individuals with knowledge, experience, patterns of thought, and values, we had best understand both the person who crafts and presents the various options as well as the often more well known individual whom he or she advises. Edward Carr, the great historiographer, wrote that "Before you study the history, study the historian.... Before you study the historian, study his historical and social environment."[3] In chapter 4 I present a set of anecdotes that suggest that Carr's dictum applies as forcefully to the study of policies and of the policy process as it does to history. The background, experience, and values of the policy maker and adviser influence the choice of words and the range of options presented.

Sometimes one has the opportunity to sense how an individual might approach a policy decision by observing that person's pattern of thought and instinctive reaction to words and events. Sometimes one can learn whether the adviser has a breadth of perspective that would enable an appreciation of the necessarily limited experience that a single individual can possess and, as a consequence, the contribution that others with different backgrounds and experiences might make to the deliberations. While not providing a conclusive template with which to assess future decisions and choices, past behavior, attitudes, and perspective may provide relevant and useful information. This chapter reminds us that in assessing policy and policy options we need to know as much as possible about the background and attitudes of those who craft policy.

The fifth chapter uses various stories to highlight the importance of the context within which the policy options are developed. Each of the anecdotes illuminates a different and important aspect of policy development. The reader will find a discussion of the importance of defining the "target" population for whom the policy is being advanced. How does one balance one's responsibility to the abstract greater society against the more visible smaller group with whom one is acquainted? Two stories will illustrate the importance of understanding the political world in which policy decisions are made, how it is that "good economics" may be trumped by important and valid political considerations and why one can be led astray if one assumes that everyone thinks and behaves as a presumed rational economist would. A final story rounds out this chapter. It reminds us that one should not be enamored of technological and overly complex solutions to problems since, on occasion, even the most difficult issues are best addressed with "simple" solutions, perhaps involving minor redefinitions of the problem.

The book closes with an epilogue which tells of an important incident in the development of President Johnson's War on Poverty. It is recounted in order to remind the reader that policy is developed by individuals, that many of these individuals are staff members who do not carry recognizable or exalted titles, and whose tasks, though important, most often do not involve a crisis or emergency. Nevertheless, the occasion may arise when their presence and commitment makes a substantial difference in the development of government policy, when things would be far different had they not been dedicated to public service. It is important to recognize that none of us knows when the opportunity to make a difference will arise, but we can be assured that it will. For some it will be in government, for others in the private sector, and for still others with family and friends. The epilogue may encourage us to recognize such occasions.

The reader will discover that many, but not all, the stories I tell come out of the health field. This is not surprising since most of my professional activities over the last forty-plus years have involved health policy matters. The events I participated in and that may have led to a story and a lesson most often took place in and were related to the medical world. Nevertheless, even while medical and health care policy have their own and unique characteristics—as do housing, transportation, education, libraries, the arts, and so on through every sector—they are part of a broader fabric which I would term social policy.

The lessons learned about health care policy development are generalizable and can be applied in other arenas as well. It is true that those especially interested in health policy may find specific examples taken from that field which may illuminate their area of interest and be directly applicable to their concerns. That, however, does not negate the potential applicability of the general lesson derived from a particular health care anecdote to other fields of policy. In that sense, the stories and the lessons, though drawn largely from one field, speak to policy development issues found in many areas.

Earlier I wrote that in studying policy it is important to understand the policy maker and adviser. I believe it is also true that in reading my narrative and stories it would be helpful to know something about the story teller. I have already referred to my interest in policy and to the influence of the household in which I was raised. There will be more "biographical notes" scattered through the later chapters. Here I would acquaint the reader with the genesis of this book, how it is that I came to rely on anecdotes as the vehicle for my observations about the role of the adviser in forming policy. Why stories?

As a young child every night—or so it seems to me now—when I went to bed my father would say "let me tell you a story" and then recount a fictional tale he had made up about one or another event in the life of two imaginary small children, Natashka and Patashka. At other times he would read me a narrative poem he had written. I have evidence that my memory is not playing tricks on me: he transcribed many of the poems and stories—the first entry was when I was not quite two years old—in a tiny handwriting in an exceedingly small diary a little over two by four inches which I still cherish eight decades later. The stories and poems were entertaining. They also were pointed and educational. They had a moral dimension and behavioral imperative. Call them "stories or poems"; call them "lessons," or as a colleague termed them: "parables."

Many years later I realized that, almost without my knowing it, I had adopted the story, the anecdote, as a way of illustrating a point, as a device to make an abstract idea more concrete. I had taken the story/poem/lesson format of my childhood days into the classroom and other settings and used it, not to entertain, but to invite students, colleagues, friends to think a bit more and perhaps in a different way about the subject at hand. There was an important difference, however: the stories I recounted were not fictional. I had observed the events I told about and most often had been a participant. Importantly, though I played a part in them, they were not stories about me. Rather, they were stories that attempted to illustrate an idea, some larger point that was relevant to the experience of the listener.

Educated as an economist, I had read Adam Smith's *An Inquiry into the Causes and Nature of the Wealth of Nations.* Perhaps now that I was a teacher, I was modeling my presentations after Smith's detailed description of a real world pin factory and his "translation" of these observations into a discussion of the consequent increase in productivity associated with the division of labor. I wanted to present inferences drawn from observation and/or from stories describing events to which the listener could relate. The story format was not used only in the classroom. It became so much a part of me that my sister-in-law began to doubt that some of the events I spoke of had actually occurred. Believing I had made them up to drive a point home, she would turn to my wife for corroboration: "Did that really happen?"

The anecdotes that follow most often involve behavior, choices, and decisions, but they are not always presented with guidelines that would determine which of the possible decisions are "correct" and which might be "incorrect." Many of the stories are of events that have no right or wrong and raise issues to which reasonable people may respond differently and on which they would disagree. The reader who hopes that I will present a formula to determine which of the numerous policy options is the one to be selected will be disappointed. Often, the stories I will tell and the points they are designed to illustrate are about a quest for balance between competing and contrasting approaches. Since that is the case, I have tried not to hector or badger the reader with strident words that might imply there is only one correct or moral way to see the problem presented.

Nevertheless, in telling many of the stories I do present my point of view. Perhaps, I do so because of my reaction to an incident which took place in the fall of 1952 when, as a young lecturer, I was teaching my first course in economics. Students had asked that I spend one class session presenting and commenting on the different economic proposals of the two presidential candidates, General Dwight Eisenhower and Governor Adlai Stevenson and I did so. At the end of the hour, after reminding the students that one's vote was properly based on many considerations, I asked that, assuming that economics were all I cared about, how many of them believed I would vote for Ike and how many for Adlai. I was thrilled that the class split eighteen to seventeen in their judgment of my preference. I concluded that though I had a strong preference for one of the candidates I had obviously made a most objective presentation.

Over the years, as I spent more hours in the classroom, I came to realize that the teachers I remembered with respect and affection and from whom I learned the most had strong views which they presented and with which they invited us to argue. We knew where they stood and argue we did. Importantly, they were fair in presenting all points of view, but did not assume a posture of neutrality that might have made their presentation bland. In 1952, I had apparently presented the issues separating Eisenhower and Stevenson fairly, but I suspect that my presentation may have been less than engaging. I see no virtue in repeating that experience. When I have a clear point of view the reader will know it and there will be no "hidden agenda."

1

The Time to Change the Rules is Before the Game Begins

On the one hand, there's an expansive view that holds that we live in a society with many—and often conflicting—values. On the other hand, there's a more constrained view that claims that we live in an economy where all that's required of us in order to make the "right" choice is a calculus of the benefits and costs of our options. Obviously, our policy debates are not only about "technical solutions to technical problems," but about values. The progressivity of the tax code, the choice between expanding federal aid to elementary and secondary schools, expanding Medicaid, and lowering taxes—these are only a few examples of how values impinge on policy. So, too, when a hospital proposes to close a service that brings uninsured patients to the emergency room on which it loses money. So, as well, when a parent makes a great economic sacrifice to help a son or daughter attend a more expensive college because it may provide a "richer" college experience. All these involve values that go beyond the purely economic.

These matters arose in the course of lengthy discussions about the first book I wrote.

In a sense writing that book, *The Economics of Mental Illness*,[1] involved an accident: I had not been especially interested in mental illness or in the economics of a disease or health condition. It is true that I had wandered into the field of health economics, though it is fair to say that at that time it wasn't a field at all, more like a small patch. But that, too, had been an accident. Let me amplify a bit on my professional development and its relationship both to the book, the issues raised therein, and its policy implications.

I attended high school and the first year of college in Bridgeport, Connecticut. When my parents moved to Baltimore, I applied as a transfer student to Johns Hopkins. I suspect I was accepted in spite of Hopkins' well-known discrimination against Jewish applicants because, as an all-male school, the impact of the World War II draft had left the university with only a few students, largely those in a V-12 training program for prospective naval officers. I completed two-thirds of my sophomore year and entered the Navy shortly after turning eighteen. In 1946, I returned to Hopkins under the G.I. Bill of Rights which paid for my tuition, books, and supplies, and provided a monthly cash stipend. Undoubtedly it was then and still remains the federal government's most effective human resource investment. During my service as an enlisted man on a destroyer I had ample time to contemplate my chemistry lab technique and wisely concluded that chemical engineering, my intended major, was not where I belonged. I searched for a new major with few departmental requirements so that I would be able to fill my schedule with courses such as American literature, economics, political science, two years of language, which were required to graduate in the Faculty of Arts and Sciences. Though I was not particularly interested or, as it turned out, especially able in mathematics, it met my pragmatic needs and became my major.

I took a maximum number of courses in the department of political economy, the discipline that in most colleges was labeled "economics." Having grown up during the Great Depression I was drawn to the subject by the belief that economics dealt with such issues as the distribution of income, employment and unemployment, the role of unions, and economic justice. Though, the Hopkins curriculum was heavily oriented toward pure theory with little attention to economic institutions and applied issues and in that sense failed to meet my expectations, I soon found that knowing some math when others knew less helped me immensely. While my limitations as a mathematician were many, the adage that in the country of the blind the one-eyed man is king helped me receive a fellowship to enter Hopkins' graduate department of political economy.

The Hopkins department had a superb faculty and a very small enrollment: only as many students—something in the order of twenty—as there were desks in the library stacks. We received an exceedingly rich grounding in economics theory as well as in history of economic thought, methodology, philosophy, history, and political science—at the time Hopkins did not yet have a sociology department. We were educated, not trained and learned to think as economists, that is, to ask a set of different questions than are asked by persons in the other social science disciplines and to be sensitive to a set of variables some of which others might overlook. Hopkins' strong liberal arts traditions meant that we were encouraged to respect colleagues in other disciplines who, because of their education, studied the very matters and factors we might ignore.

When it came time to select a dissertation topic I found that I was torn between emotion and reason, between heart and mind. Emotionally, I wanted to study something in "the real world," something that related to people, something that was "important" and dealt with policy. My horizons, however, were limited by what I knew—and whose internal logic I found attractive—and that was abstract theory. The issue was resolved when, by good fortune, I was referred to a Hopkins faculty member who suggested that I might find a meaningful topic combining my interest in theory and in something affecting real people somewhere in the field of health care: say, for example, the way physicians determined the price of medical services or the monopolistic power of hospitals.

That is how it was that I drifted into the health field. Of course, there were many steps along the way: a fellowship in the Welch Medical Library at Hopkins enabled me to read and think about relationships between economics and medicine, experience analyzing health manpower issues for the Commission on the Health Care Needs of the Nation that had been created by President Truman, an appointment at the University of North Carolina (Chapel Hill) in both the economics department and the program planning section of the Division of Health Affairs, and the completion of my dissertation on economic factors influencing the choice of location by physicians. Even so, over time I drifted away from health care issues.

If the entrance into health economics was the first "accident," the return to the field came as the result of the second one. In 1956, I was asked whether I would be interested in writing a book on the economics of mental illness for the Joint Commission on Mental Illness and Health, a private body, with partial funding from the federal government, which would conduct a wide-ranging examination of mental health in the United States. The fact that that there were no "specifications" and that I would be given complete freedom to define the inquiry as I saw fit was intriguing and I agreed to undertake the project.

I concluded that in structuring the study I might make a contribution by redefining the term "cost" as in "cost of mental illness" from the traditional accounting entry to one with greater economic content. Instead of asking how much was being spent to treat and prevent mental illness, I would determine the nature and size of its impact on the American economy. After all, that too was a "cost." Perhaps this quest for precision was the result of Fritz Machlup's influence. He was known for his interest in economic terminology: he had discovered thirty-four different definitions for "forced savings" in the economics literature and had demonstrated the confusion that resulted when authors used the term without recognizing its different meanings. His classic lecture on "elasticity of demand" distinguished the concept as seen by the seller from that as seen by the buyer and by other participants in the economic drama. It may well be, therefore, that as I thought about the costs of mental illness I realized—as will be discussed in a later chapter—that the term "cost" could mean many different things.

The book, *The Economics of Mental Illness*, documented what I called the "direct costs" of the condition, the money spent on treatment, and the "indirect costs" the loss of production, to the American economy. The measurement of the indirect costs required the kind of analytical economics I had studied: the choice of an appropriate discount rate, the necessary adjustment for unemployment, and so forth. Clearly, mental illness was much more costly than appeared at first blush, that is by simply totaling expenditures on its treatment and prevention. Because it had a large unfavorable impact on America's GNP I ended the book with the statement that the question "Can we afford to treat mental illness?" should be rephrased "Can we afford not to?"

There were a number of reasons that that question, which passed a rhetorical test and which implied a particular answer, was ill-phrased. The first was the use of the word "afford." The term is ambiguous at best and misleading at worst. As will be discussed later in this volume, as a nation we can "afford" all sorts of things if we choose to give up some other things. The second was that I had not conducted a benefit-cost analysis and, therefore, had no information on the expenditures that might be needed to prevent and, that failing, to alter the condition. The loss to the GNP was measured; the resources required to treat mental illness and negate that loss were not. Thus, I provided no information on how much we might have to give up in order to treat mental illness. Nevertheless, my question presumed a certain answer.

In my judgment, the third problem—which I did not recognize at the time—was even more basic. It lies at the heart of the matter and is part of the reason for my emphasis on the need for the policy maker and adviser to remember that "economics isn't everything" and that we all have deeply held values that extend beyond those of the economic calculus. The way I posed the question implied that the economic calculus should be compelling: mental illness was lowering GNP and, therefore, we ought to do something about it. Given its economic costs and damage could we "afford not to?" That perspective provoked lengthy arguments with my father. He was "offended" by the notion that somehow I was saying, or at least implying, that we ought to intervene because of the economic considerations. He argued we ought to intervene because human beings were suffering, because we ought to behave decently and compassionately and that meant helping human beings in distress. I argued that he was right in believing and stating that we should offer help, but wasn't it nice that that also made economic sense, that there was an economic justification for "doing good." It seemed to me that I had strengthened the argument for intervention. If there were people whose ability to make empathetic responses was underdeveloped I could appeal to their willingness to employ economic criteria to guide behavior.

My father was not satisfied. "What," he wondered, "if the economics had turned out differently, what if it cost so much to cure the problem that it was a bad "investment?" He didn't, but could have questioned the values implied by the GNP numbers and the way the loss in economic production was measured. Suppose that most of the mentally ill were female and not in the labor force, as was the case at that time, and, therefore, not adding that much to the Gross National Product which, focusing on paid labor, did not include the value of unpaid household labor? Suppose most of the mentally ill had been "unproductive" retirees? Did that make mental illness "less important?" Did my work imply that if we couldn't treat everyone we should treat those who in the past had and in the future would earn the highest salaries and wages because they would contribute more to the GNP? Did their higher pay mean they were the most productive members of society and, if so, did that really make them more "valuable"? What happens to the poet, the priest who took a vow of poverty, the janitor in a society that measures worth in that way? What happened to my economic argument under those conditions? Are some people "worth" more than others and, if so, is their worth to be measured in economic terms? What would I have done with my research if the answers I obtained turned out to be "wrong," that is at variance with my non-economic value system?

These were and are non-trivial questions. As I write I am aware of the *Boston Globe* headline on an article published August 5, 2007, "The Downside of Diversity: A Harvard Political Scientist Finds That Diversity Hurts Civic Life. What Happens When a Liberal Scholar Unearths an Inconvenient Truth?"[2] When my father asked me, a liberal scholar, essentially the same question my answer was that I could not falsify data and make up a different set of numbers. What was found was found. But, and this was an important part of my answer then even if it would no longer be so, I would not consider it incumbent to publish the results.

I have concluded that just as self-censorship hardly suffices in general, so too self-censorship after one has completed the research cannot be condoned in the world of scholarship. One cannot say, "let's play a game, but count the results only if I win." Nevertheless, at the time my answer seemed to be sufficient. It might not be acceptable economic scholarship, but I believed it might make for what I felt was good social policy.

Over the years following the late 1950s the field of health economics and the role of economists in the arena of health care have expanded significantly. This was especially the case as the health sector grew both in employment and in expenditures with the enactment of Medicare and Medicaid in 1965 and their implementation in 1966. Further expansion of what has come to be called "health services research" took place when, under President Johnson, the federal government, including the Department of Health, Education, and Welfare (the precursor to today's Department of Health and Human Services and Department of Education) adopted a program budgeting approach and began to emphasize deeper analysis of government programs. The increased attention to program analysis and evaluation included a richer understanding of the resources devoted to various endeavors and of the actual outcomes, outputs, and results of the programs in question. Often this meant undertaking benefit-cost analysis and formal attempts to compare program benefits in all their richness with program costs. Economists knew how to undertake such studies.

There is little question that analysts were aware of the limitations of their analyses, though one sometimes wondered whether that was as true of the policy makers they served. They did not have all the data necessary to capture the full range of benefits or to translate them appropriately into dollar terms nor were they able to measure all of the costs since some (as for example, pollution or the destruction of areas of scenic value) did not enter into the market economy. Thus, in addition to presenting the formal numeric findings, there often were long footnotes that pointed out the limitation of the quantified results. One may wonder about the potential misuse of the numbers given their appearance of precision even if the footnotes that tried to say, "Don't rely too heavily on these results" were eloquently written. Let us assume, however, that all the cautions were observed. There still remained the question: should social policy be guided by this kind of economic analysis? Was my father wrong in somehow feeling offended if not by the crassness of the calculation, then by the uses to which it might be put?

This question was driven home to me when I wrote a paper for a conference of pediatricians that tried to explain what benefit-cost

analysis was about, the way economists might think about balancing utilities at the margin, and the need to search for the program
that would yield the highest ratio of benefits to costs. I realized that
social policy demanded more than the maximization of production
and of the GNP. What if a larger payoff to future GNP would be
generated if more educational funds were invested in schools and
programs for those educationally advantaged (that is, for the best
students in the best schools) as compared with investments in Head
Start programs and in further efforts to raise those youngsters found
at the bottom of the educational ladder. Economic policy called for
programs that would maximize production; social policy called for
programs that would attempt to achieve greater equity and minimize
disparities. After all, a society that places a value on what might
be called "social cohesion" might very well prefer a society with
a somewhat lower GNP per capita, but with greater equality to a
society with a higher GNP, but with much wider income disparities. The wealthy person who must walk carefully in order to step
over the homeless who sleep on warm sidewalk grates might well
prefer an educational policy that raises others' skills and income
even if that comes at his expense.

If the policy adviser rejects "running the numbers" and pub-
lishing them only if they fit her or his value system or if they are
presented while ineffectually urging and even insisting that they
not be used in making decisions, what alternative course of action
can be pursued? Can one "play the game" according to a set of
rules and then, if the result isn't to one's liking call for a change
of rules? No, rules should be changed before the game is played,
not after it is over. The proper response for someone in a situation
in which he or she believes the rules are incomplete or incorrect
is not to play the game. The new "rules" need to include ways to
take account of such "values" as equity, a sharing of the benefits of
economic growth that is designed to reduce inequalities, and ways
of incorporating an increase in "social cohesion" as an important
potential benefit.

The policy maker evades his or her responsibility with the argument that the "problem" I raise is a non-problem because if, as
the economic analysis indicates, the gains to the "winners" exceed

the losses to the "losers" all that is needed is to develop ways to share these greater gains, that is to compensate the losers and still have some gains left over. The fact that problems of this sort can be solved does not mean that they will be solved. The record of failure, in fact, is a long one. We have not effectively dealt with similar kinds of problems that we encounter: the building of a new runway accommodating more flights and of benefit to the greater community, but which adds to the noise pollution for close by residents; the problem faced by so many organizations and enterprises that elicit the response, "not in my back yard" when they attempt to expand; the frictions that arise in conjunction with free trade and NAFTA policies which help many Americans but hurt others.

One can object to my formulation. I have a colleague who argues that it is better to know something than to know nothing and that my unwillingness to do this kind of analysis results in knowing nothing. There is some merit to that way of looking at the problem. Yet, I have come to believe that there is a greater danger associated with knowing something, but thinking that and behaving as if one knows enough and even everything.

The problem of overemphasis on quantitative rigor and economic analysis in evaluation of potential federal programs is real and pervasive. Some months after President Johnson issued his executive order calling on all departments of the government to institute program budgeting and more rigorous analysis of the benefits and costs of federal programs I was asked to join a task force ("Program Analysis Group: 5; Comprehensive Health Care for Children") that the Department of Health, Education, and Welfare had established in an effort to respond to the president's desire to develop a child health program. The task force was asked to think through the issues, set priorities, and recommend the characteristics of a program. It was to define the goals and evaluate the costs of "alternative packages of programs" that might be designed to attain those goals. The directive to the task force also stated that "Evaluation of the effectiveness of the many current Federal programs to improve child health is also essential." Given the president's executive order, the program had to be justified as meeting cost-benefit criteria.

Under the guidance of the physician chairman, the deliberations emphasized the early detection of genetic and other early childhood problems that might affect future labor force participation and productivity and that, if dealt with at an early stage, could reverse potential negative outcomes and thus increase potential future output. There was much discussion of possible conditions and of potential appropriate interventions. The discussions were interesting and all participants were more than compassionate. Nevertheless, I was troubled and after attending a few meetings that seemed to approach the problem in the same analytic manner that was increasingly constrained by the lack of the data required to "prove" the benefit-cost relationship, I spoke up in an effort to redirect our approach.

> What about the following. Don't we care about the child who is sick and spends the night crying and tossing and turning and whose parents are up all night, worried, concerned, holding the child and trying to sooth it. The illness is self limiting and everything will be fine in a week or so and there will be no prolonged after affects. Still, what if we could create a program that provided appropriate health care and medication such that the child would recover in four days? The benefits of that program would be limited to an increase in (unmeasured) well being: a few days and nights with less pain, less crying, and more sleep. Perhaps not losing as much sleep, the parents would be a bit more productive, but even that would be minimal at best. The economy would be no stronger, but the parents' concerns would have been assuaged and the social condition would have been improved.

Everyone agreed that my imaginary problem was important and should not be ignored. But there were no data and there was no way to generate data that measured the benefit of that kind of early intervention and improvement in well-being. And certainly there was no accepted way to convert those benefits into dollars. My attempt to redirect our attention to a different kind of problem and a different kind of intervention failed. Absent the numbers, the required justification for a program was missing. Absent the required justification, the program was not part of the agenda.

Over time, policy advisers may learn how to incorporate nontraditional variables into their analyses and thus have a much richer measure of "progress" than the increase in the nation's GDP.

Over time, they may learn how to control their hubris about how much they know and may come to recognize that modesty about how well they can measure and analyze non-economic measures is called for. Till those days come, I fear that a narrow economic approach that often rests on mathematic and statistical techniques that policy makers may not understand and, therefore, may not question, may—unless policy advisers are diligent in their effort to be broad ranging and unashamed at adding "values" to their discourse—be more powerful than is appropriate.

A long time ago, in 1974, I appeared on an "ABC News Closeup" that examined "Children: A Case of Neglect." The program dealt with the failures of the Nixon administration in dealing with America's dismal record regarding the health of children. I had been interviewed some weeks earlier and summarized what I believed by saying what became the closing remarks of the documentary: "Frankly, I'm tired of the argument that we ought to do these things because they are good economic investments. I think we ought to do these things because we ought to be humane, and we ought to be decent. I would like to think we are a decent people." My father and I argued in 1959. By 1974 it was evident he had won the debate.

Nevertheless, policy analysts and the public who follow policy debates need and deserve a stronger answer than one that rests on impatience. How do we assure that we are not unduly influenced by incomplete analyses which appear to be precise and which, because of the influence of quantification may carry great and undue weight? How can we make certain that concepts that cannot easily be measured, concepts such as social solidarity or equity, enter appropriately into the decision process? How do we select the weights that we attach to the variables that reflect our social preferences? Surely the answers are not clear. What is clear, however, is that the questions need to be debated and that the policy adviser need not be "embarrassed" at being considered "soft" when he or she raises them.

2

The Meaning and Influence of Words

Words, Attitudes, and Behavior

Policy advice is provided orally, by memoranda, in handwritten notes, and nicely bound print-outs. Whatever the medium, the ideas are transmitted through words, and we are all aware that the choice of words and the way they are put together makes a difference. If well chosen, they set a context, convey a meaning, and help in guiding the listener's or the reader's understanding. That is true in poetry, novels, and drama and helps to distinguish great writing from the pedestrian and dross. All of us also recognize that words may be chosen in order to influence behavior as, for example, in advertising, sloganeering, descriptions on menus and reviews of wines, as well as other matters that at the extreme border on fiction at worst and exaggeration at best.

That words make a difference is also true in non-fiction. Consider the power of great orations, Edward R. Murrow's reports from London before and during the Second World War, the articles by journalists who succeed in enlightening us about Supreme Court decisions or in conveying the impact of powerful hurricanes and devastating fires, and in describing the joys associated with triumph and the crushing aspects of defeat. There may be fewer examples of great writing or even of careful consideration of language and choice of words in the articles, monographs, and books written by academics, especially if they are written for other academics. Yet we find scholars in every discipline—for example, John Kenneth Galbraith in economics—who provide examples of careful and great writing. Indeed, that is even true of policy materials prepared for presidents and other government officials as, for example, was the case with the memoranda prepared by Theodore Sorenson, Walter Heller, and Daniel Patrick Moynihan.

Words can be effective in capturing attention and, on occasion, in putting arguments into the sorts of slogans that, by coloring and evoking emotional reactions, help determine, crystallize, and perhaps polarize the nature of disputes and that, regrettably, may preclude exploration of the "grey" areas that lie between the black and white dichotomies. Thus, "right to work" is a more politically effective way to cast an argument than "no union shop allowed." Who after all can be opposed to the "right to work?" Of course, that is not what the slogan is about nor is that the underlying issue, but… So, too, with the "right to life" which is not a slogan that relates to capital punishment or to the life of the pregnant woman when that right intersects with issues around abortion. The "the right to life" phrase is designed to be so compelling that it would preclude nuanced discussion of issues. Similarly, who among us would favor a "death tax" even though one might support estate taxation? Consider how different the debate about health care reform might be if propents of a program called "single-payer" had used the phrase "Medicare for all." The former is an unfamiliar term and does not provide an inuitive understanding of the change sought; the latter describes a program with which many Americans have intersected and which is both liked and supported. The former conjures up the treat of the unknown; the latter is familiar and acceptable. Consider, as well, how economic debates are shaped by calling something a "bailout" rather than a "loan" or "economic stimulus," by the word "nationalization" rather than "temporary receivership." Recently I saw an effort—thus far largely unsuccessful—to replace the terms "downsizing" by "rightsizing" and "layoff" by "operations improvement." Those concerned with downsizings, persons who are distressed at the human toll of layoffs and who support actions to mitigate their impact on individuals, families, and communities might well be encouraged to ignore such matters by the term's bland repackaging. After all, we need not be concerned with rightsizing and operations improvement since such actions surely must lead to favorable outcomes that are in the national interest.

Sloganeering has entered into the legislative domain. In recent years the Republican majority in Congress had taken to adding "public relations" descriptors to the otherwise "dull" numbering or naming system to proposed legislation. Thus: the "U.S.A. Patriot Act" (itself an acronym for "Uniting and Strengthening America by Providing Appropriate Tools Required to Intercept and Obstruct Terrorism Act of 2001," the "No Child Left Behind Act", and the "Partial-Birth Abortion Ban Act." Surely these have more of a ring to them than "Anti-terrorism Act of 2001," "Amendments to the Elementary and Secondary Education Act" (landmark legislation enacted during President Johnson's administration), or "Late-term Abortion Ban Act" or, though not quite synonymous, "Intact Dilation and Extraction Act." Surely it was easier to engage citizens and rally support for legislation entitled "Medicare Prescription Drug, Improvement, and Modernization Act" than for "2003 Medicare Amendments." We are a long way from such descriptors as "The Social Security Act," or "Title XVIII and Title XIX" of the Social Security Act which we know as Medicare and Medicaid respectively. The legislation outlawing discrimination in educational programs and activities receiving federal funds is known quite simply as "Title IX" (of the Education Amendments of 1972). Perhaps it would have created less resistance had it had a more super-charged advertising slogan descriptor than its official—and now forgotten—name: the "Patsy T. Mink Equal Opportunity in Education Act."

Yes, words are important: they affect attitudes and, in turn, attitudes affect behavior. The policy advisor must choose her or his language with care. What she may consider a mere descriptor that presumably carries no particular implication may turn out not to be "neutral," but consciously or unconsciously to represent a point of view. Examples of such terminology abound. Some of the newer language of medicine has that characteristic. It changes attitudes and relationships and, in my judgment, does so for the worse. Thus, the quite respectable older term "physician" is often replaced by "producer" even as the "patient" has become a "consumer." These newer, yet familiar and common terms carried over from economic discourse, are part of the economist's language. Undoubtedly they were viewed as value-free, neutral, and innocuous.

I have come to believe that economists were mistaken. I have come to understand why it was that on one occasion when I used these terms in a discussion, Julius Krevans, the then chancellor of the University of California (San Francisco), brought his fist down so forcefully on the conference table that he startled all participants and, appropriately, got their attention. He told us that he had a Peter Pan-like image of the world and that every time I used the terms "producer" and "consumer" rather than "physician" and "patient," "one more good fairy died and when they were all gone there will be no humanity left in medicine."[1] At the time I disagreed, but I have come to believe he was correct. Words help define relationships and the relationship between the producer and the consumer, a relationship akin to that found in many areas of commerce, is not what we patients desire when we come to our physician.

We should be clear, however, that economists do not have a monopoly on the fault and danger I describe. One should be as concerned with the language physicians and others use as with that which economists employ. Some minutes after invoking the Peter Pan image and the decline of humanity in medicine, Dr. Krevans employed the phrase "patient compliance." To me the phrase smacked of the criminal justice system. It was my turn to object that the relationship implied by the words "compliance" and "compliant" did not encompass my definition—and I hoped not his—of "humanity in medicine." We reached a truce, a truce we have observed, at least in each other's presence: each would avoid the words at issue. Words are important: they change attitudes and attitudes affect behavior, the way I view my physician and the way he views me.

Yes, we do want certain things that consumers want and that are not traditionally found in the doctor-patient relationship. Many of us do want more information than often was provided in the past; we do want to be involved in and many individuals—perhaps especially younger adults—want to be in control of the decision-making process. After all, our tastes and values, the weights we assign to different variables, may differ from those embodied in the physician's culture and attitudes. We want to be treated without the arrogance sometimes exhibited by "experts" who convey their findings and recommendations in a language to which we are not privy. Many of the things are characteristics we expect to find in our relationships as consumers in other sectors of the economy. Nevertheless, that does not negate or substitute for important elements in the traditional doctor-patient relationship. The physician is not just another salesman; medical care is not the same as soap or orange juice. Her or his office is not a used car lot.

Many if not most policy advisers, including economists, are convinced of their "objectivity" and seem unaware of and would dispute the idea that their language embodies or implies a set of relationships that are defined by and help define a value system. Yet I would argue that their language is far from value free and neutral. Significant losses may be incurred when their patterns of thought, expressed as they are through words, is carried over to other fields where words may have other meanings. I do not refer to technical words or disciplinary jargon; it is not the fact that "rent" means one thing to economists and quite another to the lay person. Such words may cause confusion, but no more than that. I refer to loss. That is the case, for example, when the physician in a hospital radiology department finds that she and her department are viewed and described as "profit centers" and comes to feel and to behave differently in response to the implicit signal the words convey. When the hospital becomes part of the "hospital industry" rather than of the "hospital sector" it has moved closer to becoming the "hospital business."

"Running the not-for-profit hospital like a business"—of course one may wonder whether the presumption that our for-profit business enterprises are run efficiently is accurate—may start out stressing buying pencils, scalpels, and pharmaceuticals at lower prices, and turning out the lights in unoccupied rooms. There is the danger, however, that over time that hospital will begin to view itself as an organization with business norms on pricing, advertising, and selection of "customers" as well. "Buy cheap and sell dear" has been a business norm; it is not and should not be the health care institution's goal and purpose. On some occasions reducing quality in order to reduce price and increase market share may yield higher profits to the retailer; it is not what patients are looking for.

Of course, it is cumbersome for not-for-profit hospitals to report that their "operating income exceeded operating expenses." The shorthand "we made a profit" is much simpler. Surely, that is part of the reason that newspapers apply the "profit and loss" terminology in reporting on hospital and other not-for-profit health care activities. The other part of the reason, however, is that far too often that is the very description that hospital officials use. I know, because I fought a losing battle over many years in trying to get a hospital vice president for finance not to use the term "profit" in reporting the hospital's financial status to the board of trustees. Everyone agreed with me whenever I raised the issue, but by the next meeting the ubiquitous term "profit" had again appeared. I suggested that the choice of words has consequences in the way the institution views itself and, as well, in the way it is viewed by others. I felt it was no accident that a number of state attorneys general, including the one for Massachusetts where the hospital was located had turned to not-for-profits who reported how profitable they were and had asked that they justify their tax-exempt status and report what "community benefits"—the presumed justification for their not-for-profit status—they provided. One cannot boast about profits in reporting to the *Boston Globe* and eschew the term when speaking to the attorney general who surely had read the morning newspaper.

Words make a difference. Our attitudes are colored by the words that we and other choose. "Payment" and "reimbursement" for medical care conjure up different images: the former implies a negotiated and agreed upon fee and offers the potential for "profit." The latter implies mere reimbursing the hospital for its costs, though the definition of what is included in costs is an important and often divisive matter. The chairman of the committee which in 1965-1966 drew up the regulations that stated what could and what could not be considered and counted as costs (e.g., the annual golf tournament, the summer "day at the races," the lobster bake, and the Christmas party) told me that there were days on which he felt that he alone was standing between the American Hospital Association and the gold in Fort Knox. Nevertheless, "reimbursement," the word used in Medicare payments to hospitals, is often viewed as negating profits and making them unlikely if not impossible.

"Premiums" are not the same as "taxes"; the latter carry a government and, for many, an onerous connotation while the former seem to imply choice and voluntary payments in the private market—unless, of course, one is required to purchase insurance. The Medicare Part B premium is not a tax, though in many respects it passes the tax test: it walks like a tax and quacks quite like a tax, and one might appropriately call it a tax. That does not make it "bad." "Beneficiaries," the term used to describe individuals who receive Social Security payments and who are covered by Medicare are not the same as "recipients," the term used to classify individuals on welfare and who are receiving Medicaid assistance. The beneficiary has earned—both literally and figuratively—the benefit; the recipient receives his support because of our largess and the milk of human kindness, and they and we are aware that on occasion milk may curdle. The very choice of language used in government tables and charts about "beneficiaries" and "recipients" is revealing.

Those who advise on policy matters understand the power of words and the fact that certain words elicit strong and often emotional responses. It is no accident that annual budget debates in Washington and many state capitals involve the word "afford" as in "we can't afford that program" and the word "cut" as in "that represents a cut in expenditures." The use of the word "afford" is most problematic since what one really means when one says "we can't afford" is that, within a given total budget, one elects not to spend money on a particular activity, but on some other. A complete statement would make it clear that one presumably cannot "afford" ABC because—with a fixed budget—one has chosen to allocate resources for something else, say XYZ, in preference to the particular matter that we "can't afford." When government officials say they can't afford something they really mean that they elect not to finance that "something" by reducing other expenditures and that they do not favor actions that would increase tax revenues and make the new expenditure possible.

The word "cut" also turns out to require more specificity. Citizens are entitled to be confused when they hear proponents of a particular program complain that it has been cut even as they read that its appropriations have increased. The explanation lies in the meaning of the term "cut." It may be that expenditures are increasing but are not keeping up with inflation and, thus, in purchasing power. As a consequence, in real terms there is a cut. Perhaps the appropriation—though growing—represents a decline in funds available per affected individual because the growth does not keep up with the expansion of the eligible population. The affected persons will experience a cut. "Cuts" may mean that though more dollars are appropriated for the program activity, the appropriation falls short of previously announced goals or legislative authorizations; perhaps fewer dollars have been appropriated than the president, governor, or chief executive requested. In a partisan debate the words "afford" and "cut" are likely to be invoked as rhetorical devices rather than as phrases designed to illuminate and inform discourse.

One may wish that things were different, that language would be employed only to illuminate. Or would we? One is reminded of Ed Murrow's phrase about Winston Churchill, "Now the hour had come for him to mobilize the English language, and send it into battle, a spearhead of hope for Britain and the world."[2] Would we have preferred a more prosaic, less rhetorical, and blander Churchill? Hardly. In any case, there is no question that even if we wished that language would not be used and words would not be chosen in order to win policy debates—that such debates be resolved solely by analytical criteria invoked by rational actors (say, computers programmed by other computers)—the wish would not be fulfilled. All that we can ask for is that our allies and opponents not do violence to the facts and that we be on guard against the influence of emotional words and incomplete arguments.

Many years ago I received a mailing from an investment firm. It told me that it really cared about my "retirement future." In that context it informed me that I spent one-third of my time "working for the government." I was angered and responded that I was pleased the firm joined me in being concerned about my retirement, but that I would have preferred to receive advice, not editorial comment. I wrote, "You inform me that I have spent one-third of my time 'working for the government.' Actually, I believe I spend one-third of my time working so that my grandchildren can have schools to go to and parks to play in, The one-third of my time you tell me I spend 'working for the government' I see as working for roads without potholes and for clean water and air. When I bought a new car I never thought I was working for the Ford Motor Company—I was working to buy a new car. In just the same way, I was working to pay the taxes which buy the things that government provides." I did not receive any reply. There is a difference between the economist's term "tax burden"—surely one does not want to increase, but to reduce, a burden—and the statements by Justice Oliver Wendell Holmes, Jr. "Taxes are what we pay for a civilized society"[3] and by Franklin Delano Roosevelt "Taxes, after all, are the dues that we pay for the privileges of membership in an organized society."[4] "Burden" is not a neutral word. That, after all, is why—when preceded by "tax"—it has migrated into the realm of political discourse. That, after all, is why we do not term expenditures on food, clothing, or recreation as the food, clothing, or recreation burden.

Words that elicit emotional reactions and that are chosen for that very purpose hardly contribute to rational discussion of issues. They do not enhance the quality of public discourse and debate. It is as Francis Bacon stated: "The ill and unfit choice of words wonderfully obstructs the understanding." But, of course, some words are selected to do just that and from the point of view of the user are not at all "ill and unfit" choices.

We are sensitive to words and, perhaps, especially to unexpected use of language that forces us to take note. Sometimes that is to the good; sometimes it is not. There is no formula to tell us which changes and which words are appropriate and especially so since the same words carry different meanings depending on context. Though some members of today's Supreme Court seem to believe that the meaning of words is immutable, never changing, and what we presume they meant at one time is what they mean today, they might well consider what Justice Holmes who served on the United States Supreme Court for a full thirty years and surely respected the power, meaning, and precision of words wrote, "A word is not a crystal, transparent and unchanged; it is the skin of living thought and may vary greatly in color and content according to the circumstances and time in which it is used."[5] Absent the formula, there is only the recognition that language counts and should be treated carefully and with respect. But that's a lot.

The Impact of Unexpected Language

Sometimes the words that influence us are effective because they are unexpected. It is not the slogan at all, but the fact that one is forced to stop and consider what was said. Perhaps it is that the words are said in a particular manner, say, with passion or with humor; perhaps it is that they convey the unexpected and we are taken aback. We are forced to think. Let me describe one such occurrence and the impact it had on my research agenda. It happened some years ago when New York City was facing a budget crisis and the then mayor announced that among other initiatives to reduce duplication of services he planned to rationalize and consolidate the city's health care services. One measure called for the closing of one of the city hospitals whose disproportionally African-American patients would receive their care elsewhere. Persons in the affected neighborhood protested and rallied against the planned closure. I read about the event in the *New York Times*. A sentence quoting one of the many speakers at the most recent rally began with the words, "Mr. Mayor, you're taking away our…" At that point my reading was interrupted (perhaps the story was continued on an inside page, perhaps the phone rang). When I returned to the account I "knew" how the sentence ended: the words "health care" came to mind. Surely the protesters were accusing the mayor of taking away their health care. Thus it was a shock that the sentence that began "Mr. Mayor, you're taking away our" ended with the one word "jobs." The shock of the unanticipated word caused me to think.

It is not necessary to describe the thought processes that ensued. All of us are aware that the health sector generates employment. All of us recognize the fact that though some of the many jobs are held by health care professionals—by persons trained in health care disciplines—others are held by administrators, communications specialists, photographers, accountants, cleaning personnel, and countless others. Some of us are old enough to recall that when Medicare and Medicaid were enacted—both called for new kinds of record keeping and accountability—some wags referred to them as "The Accountants and Bookkeepers Relief Act of 1965." Nevertheless, most of the time we think of the health sector and of hospitals as delivering medical care rather than as generating employment. Thus, "You're taking away our jobs" sent a jarring message that could not be ignored. I do not know whether it caused the New York City administration to reevaluate its policy plans. I do know that a few years later it led me to join a colleague in writing a policy-oriented paper that called upon the body politic to recognize that health care cost containment efforts had important implications for workers and local economies and that "downsizing" the health care sector and closing hospital beds required that we plan and prepare for changes in the demand for labor. The unemployed practical nurse was not likely to find a job in the expanding financial sector. We need to recognize that even when the larger society benefits from health care cost containment efforts, some individuals will be negatively affected. Some of us are "winners," others are "losers." We argued that public policy needed to develop programs—job retraining, employment counseling, and income maintenance—to assist those who "lose" lest their resistance to change precludes progress. Sometimes those who think, write, or advise about policy matters need to be—and are—awakened to issues and impelled to think differently because of a phrase, a word, and even an interrupted sentence.

But thought patterns do not change alone because of words in a newspaper, a fiscal crisis, a mayoral decision, a speaker at a protest rally. Sometime in the spring, around 1970, give or take a year, my wife, older daughter age twelve or so and I were sitting in the family room in our home in Newton, Massachusetts. I do not remember what we were discussing, but at some point the twelve year old delivered a heartfelt declarative sentence: "I feel passionately about women's rights!" I burst out laughing—not a wise thing to do with anyone who is making a heartfelt statement; an exceedingly dumb thing to do to a twelve-year-old daughter whose statement begged to be taken seriously. My laughter, after all, was not about humor. It was condescending and dismissive. "Why are you laughing?" she asked. I replied that her statement struck me as odd: "You're twelve and you say you feel passionately. Surely that's a bit much for a twelve year old."

Her response was quick in coming. "If I had said 'I feel passionately about civil rights' would you have laughed or been proud of me?" Oops! I had been convinced the issue was that "passionately" was simply too strong a term for a twelve-year-old youngster. Now that hypothesis was put to the test: was my problem "passionately" or "women's rights" or, perhaps, some combination of the two. For as Karen well knew, her question answered itself. Had she said "civil rights" I would have interpreted that to mean issues related to race and wouldn't have laughed. I would have been proud of her and, truth be told, would have claimed credit for having imparted my values so successfully. Apparently therefore, I could handle the idea that twelve year olds felt "passionately." Apparently my reaction suggested that feeling passionately about civil rights was fine, something of which this parent could be proud, but women's rights could not or should not command that level of intensity. If so, what was the basis for that view?

I suppose that one might mount an argument (it needn't be compelling, just "not off the wall") that there are differences in the degree and kind of discrimination faced by women and by African-Americans in the United States. I also suppose that one could argue that how deeply one felt about injustices levied against "others" (I am concerned, I care, I feel strongly, I would sign a petition, write my congressman, donate funds, march on Washington) might depend on the kind of injustice and discrimination, the nature of the bigotry and the number of persons affected. Similarly, one might argue that a glass ceiling or wage differential is not the same as a lynching—if there be those who think otherwise they should listen to Billie Holiday singing "Strange Fruit." Yet, I do not think those or similar factors were at play in my response. I didn't parse and analyze the words; I laughed. Nor could I argue that my views were colored by the fact that my daughter's views about feminism were more self-serving than similar views about racial discrimination. After all, I did not think less of Martin Luther King than of whites who marched at Selma even though one might argue that a loosening of segregation's bonds would directly benefit the former and "only" indirectly the latter. Nor did I think more of those who, though not personally affected, supported a strike than I did of the worker on the picket line who might gain higher wages from the strike.

No, I rather think that the visceral reaction of laughter most probably revealed an attitude, a bias that I was unaware of: that passion about civil rights was appropriate and was to be commended while passion, real passion, was an overreaction to issues of feminism. I simply cannot imagine that I would have arrived at that understanding of myself and about my biases through some rational argument. I believe it took an extraordinary non-rhetorical statement and question to remind me of the relationship between civil rights and women's rights and by forcing the issue reveal deep seated attitudes and, to some—perhaps, significant—degree, acceptance of the status quo. Nor can I imagine that my (or anyone else's) view of the world, of policy issues and agendas, and of private and public decisions on a wide variety of matters, could remain unaffected when the individual is forced to confront and question very basic and, perhaps, deep seated views.

Same Words, but Different Meanings

Individual words do make a difference. They color our attitudes and responses. On occasion they are put together in a manner that increases their power and that makes the sum greater than its individual parts. But we should be clear: badly chosen words or poorly constructed phrases are not benign or mere missed opportunities to say something "better" or more persuasively. Ill-chosen words— ideas expressed in words that may be accurate, but that are less than complete and, therefore, subject to misinterpretation—may do harm to the point that one is trying to make and to the policy agenda one is trying to advance. The words may be "correct," the presentation may be a blunder. I know whereof I write.

I joined the staff of the Council of Economic Advisers (CEA)— the body charged with responsibility to advise the president on economic affairs—in the summer of 1961, only a few months after the inauguration of President Kennedy. At that time (though regrettably not today) the CEA was housed next door to the White

House in the Old Executive Office Building (now named the Eisen-hower Executive Office Building), an ornate structure built during the 1870s and 80s. At one time, when government was smaller and when security concerns were less, this remarkable building housed the State, War, and Navy departments and was open to the general public. Its offices were spacious with high ceilings and large windows. Many had marble fireplaces. The door hinges and handles were engraved (rumor had it that was true on the inside facing the wood as well as on the visible outside) with the "coat of arms" of the department of State, Navy, or War. It was a building that made both those who worked and those who visited within its walls, so proximate to the White House, feel important. Even so, the exhilaration that staff members at the Council felt when we entered the building was far more influenced by the spirit of the times, by the excitement of the new administration.

I had come to the CEA on a two year leave of absence from my position at the University of North Carolina (Chapel Hill). At the time I was contemplating a move to another university, but was hoping that I would be able to find a position somewhere in the new administration and when the offer came from what was likely to be the best place in Washington for a young economist, I went to the dean and requested leave. He expressed surprise when I told him I wanted to go to Washington: "Why? I've been there. It's hot and humid." I did not tell him about the meaning of the Liberty Bell, but blurted out that "America has been good to my parents who came here in 1923 and through them to me. If there is someone in Washington who believes I could make some contribution to my country and asks me to do so, I have to respond." I am not certain he understood, but leave was granted.

The expectation of a new direction for America (of a "New Frontier") and the desire to be part of that change motivated me and many of my colleagues who also came to Washington in 1961. For example, when the chairman of the Council, Walter Heller, invited me to join the CEA staff and asked what my university salary was, I was aware that there were real constraints on the Council budget. It had remained at the same level over the fifteen years since the CEA had been created by the Full Employment

Act in 1946. I feared that Walter might not be able to offer me a salary as high as the close to $13,000 per year I was making after adding the summer stipend and the evening teaching I was doing at North Carolina College (now North Carolina Central University) in Durham to the $9,600 I was earning at UNC. Afraid that he would be troubled about asking me to take a cut in income, I reduced the sum I quoted to Heller. I was convinced that somehow my wife and I and our four children would manage. Similarly, when I asked my close colleague and friend on the Council staff, Bob Lampman, what he was making, he told me that he didn't know. It turned out that that was not merely because he hadn't yet received a paycheck and was not aware of the nature and size of the deductions for taxes and fringes. Rather, he didn't know because he had accepted Heller's invitation without asking what the gross salary would be. He simply assumed that the chairman would make certain it would be enough to live on. Neither of us was surprised at each other's behavior. Nor, unlike the secretiveness with which salaries were treated in the university, were we embarrassed in discussing the topic. For many citizens—though, of course, not for all—1961 was a very special time; for an economist, the Council was a very special place.

The council staff members had a very close rapport. That was the result of at least four factors. The first was that a number of staff members (though neither Bob nor I) had been students of Jim Tobin of Yale, a great economist and mentor and one of the three council members. The second was that few of us, on leave from universities, were well versed in the "ways of Washington." I had the good sense to ask a friend who had worked for government and knew a lot about Washington and the individuals who worked in the various agencies, what I should do now that I was "on board" and had an office. Walter's directive provided insufficient guidance: "Go to it. You know more about your areas of responsibility than I so do what you think best." My friend told me whom to call and invite to lunch: the civil servants who knew a lot and had policy proposals languishing in file drawers, proposals they would want to share with someone who was working next door to the White House. Because so many of us at the Council were new to government and so ignorant of its ways, we relied on each other and shared information and knowledge. The virtues of cooperation dominated over those generated by competition, important as the latter was to economists.

The third factor that united us was what I might term the "we were at Iwo Jima together" syndrome. Often we worked well into the evening and during Economic Report time (just after Thanksgiving to mid-January) well into the night or early morn, day after day, seven days a week. The feeling of long hours and of tension brought us together (though we were old enough to be exquisitely aware that, in fact, this was not Iwo Jima). The fourth factor may well have been the most important. Many of us had left our academic positions and come to Washington not because we assumed that the experience would enhance our careers, though it may well have done so, or because we believed that we would all learn useful things about the formulation of public policy, though we most assuredly did. We came because of the sense of excitement that the newly elected young president had brought to Washington and to the nation and because of the aspect of public service that he articulated in his Inaugural address as in—who can dispute that words do make a difference—"And so, my fellow Americans: ask not what your country can do for you—ask what you can do for your country."

As noted, I had joined the staff of the Council of Economic Advisers at the beginning of July, 1961. That October I was a delegate to a nineteen-nation Policy Conference on Economic Growth and Investment in Education. There are three reasons I remember the event quite vividly. The first was that the conference, called by the Organization for Economic Co-operation and Development (OECD) at that time encompassing the European nations, Canada, and the United States, entailed two black tie events. I did not own a tuxedo, had never owned a tuxedo (a three-season blue suit sufficed for our wedding), and did not anticipate owning a tuxedo. But this was Washington and this, presumably, was what Washington was—at least in part—about! Thus, it seemed to make sense to purchase a tux since already in the first three and a half months after joining the Council there were two occasions that called for black tie and I was to be at the Council for two years. I went to Raleigh's clothing store, purchased a tuxedo and all the paraphernalia that goes with it, wore it to the two banquets, and waited for the deluge of invitations that would follow. Deluge? Not even a trickle. I received no other invitations. By the time I had occasion to wear black tie again many years later I found that either the tuxedo had shrunk or I had gained weight. I prefer the former explanation.

The second reason that I remember the occasion was that I prepared the address that Walter Heller, chairman of the Council, delivered at the concluding banquet. Walter was gracious enough to insert a footnote in the printed version of the address stating that he was indebted to me for assistance in preparing his remarks. Furthermore, in the address the phrase that, as drafted, had simply stated "In this connection I am reminded that…" was delivered with a change that stated, "In this connection I am reminded by Rashi Fein that…" But there was a problem: by then I had sat with the other delegates for some three days, had participated in vigorous discussion (more on that later) and social events and was known to them. Walter was not. As a consequence, a number of delegates rushed over to me after the banquet to congratulate me on the "excellent speech" that I had drafted. I am certain that Walter also received congratulatory remarks, yet the impression that I had and retained was that he was left standing alone—another case of "no good deed shall go unpunished"—while I was surrounded by well wishers. Needless to say, I was both embarrassed and troubled. Upstaging one's "boss" is not a good idea. Furthermore, whatever the quality of the speech, it was the delivery thereof—words make a difference, but the way they are delivered does so as well—that merited the kudos. I and other staff members were not surprised that in the future staff members received somewhat less public recognition for their contributions.

But it is the third remembrance that was significant. The conference was held on October 17, 1961, and when I opened up the *New York Times* on the early morning of the 18th I found an article with a series of headlines: "U.S. AIDE DENIES LAG IN TEACHERS" "Economist tells 19-Nation Parley Only Shortage Is One of Effectiveness" "DECRIES 'BABY SITTING'" "But Delegates From Europe Insist That Gap Exists—Proposals Are Offered." The first paragraph of the article identified the U.S. aide as "An economist with the President's Council of Economic Advisers." The second paragraph attached my name to that descriptor.[6] The thrill of having one's name in the *Times* was more than tempered by the story to which it was attached. What I had stated appeared to be at variance with the Kennedy administration's very public position that America faced a large shortage of teachers. I was very concerned. At the minimum I expected a severe reprimand. At the maximum I wondered whether this would effectively cost me my position. I had already submitted a memo that because of inadequate proofreading stated "millions" when it should have been "billions." Would this new and more damaging faux pas mean that I might hang around for a time, but wouldn't be given any responsible assignments, that I would not continue to be involved?

I dressed quickly and rushed to the office hoping to explain things before any of the three Council members read the article. The explanation would amplify the points that Marjorie Hunter who filed the story had included in the account. I was quoted correctly as stating, "There is no shortage of teachers, only a shortage of effective teaching." The article also stated that I had alluded to the good things the nation was doing to free good teachers from "baby-sitting" duties and cited educational television as one example. The headlines were a disaster, but the article was both accurate and balanced. Nevertheless—and this clearly was the fault of my presentation—it didn't adequately convey the ideas I had in mind. Furthermore, the article made clear that my comments had not been well received, that I was in the distinct minority and "One after another delegates from Europe complained of a serious shortage." It then referred to statements by the delegates from Denmark ("had to reduce school hours because of the teacher shortage"); Switzerland (there was an "enormous shortage" and beginning salaries in private industries were sometimes three or four times those of teachers); Italy (echoing the difficulty that government faced in competing with salaries in private industry). The delegate from the Netherlands did suggest that a few years earlier his country raised salaries, liberalized training scholarships, and offered tax relief to parents of college students and that the result of these various measures had "been remarkably good."

It was Philip Coombs, assistant secretary of state for education and cultural affairs and head of the U. S. delegation who amplified my much too terse remark that there was no teacher shortage and put it into an appropriate economic framework. He stated that he wanted to discuss "the teaching bottleneck...as distinct from the statistical number of teachers" and that he wanted to speak about actions on what he termed the supply and the demand side. Supply increases could be furthered by enlarging teacher training facilities, by raising salaries, and by recruiting married women who had left the profession. Measures to shrink the demand for teachers could involve freeing teachers to teach and "not have to help the children off with their snowsuits or erase blackboards." He noted "that the teaching profession was the only one that had failed to develop a system of division of labor between the highly trained and the assistants."

Concerned about the front-page story, I reached the office prepared to admit that my choice of words left much to be desired, but explaining that what I had meant was that we should be looking at teaching, not teachers. The economist in me wanted to recognize that even a focus on "teaching" was inadequate since "teaching" and "teachers" deal with inputs while our real concern is with output, that is, with "learning." But I knew that refinement would be ignored. I wanted to make clear that although a more precise statement might not have helped on the public relations front, I knew that at most I should have said, "We may or may not need more teachers. The way to determine that is to decide how much teaching we need and how many teachers we would need to do that teaching if teachers were relieved of the duties they now have, duties that do not require their level of education and training."

The rest of the story is simple. In one of life's ego shattering experiences I found that no one at the Council or in the White House seemed to care about what I said and the story the *New York Times* had published. Perhaps those in the Office of Education or in the teachers' unions who might have criticized me read the entire article carefully and found themselves in agreement. Perhaps it really wasn't all that important. After all, the president had already stated there was a shortage and it's what presidents not staff economists say that counts. In any case, I was aware of only two references to the event. One was in a brief note quoting the sentence that there is no shortage of teachers under the heading "Notable and Quotable" in the *Wall Street Journal*. Not surprisingly, the *Journal* was rather taken with the idea that this "U.S. Aide" disagreed with President Kennedy and had revealed the truth. The second was in an editorial in the *Dallas Morning News* which also praised the fact that I took a position "in direct contrast to the propaganda from the Kennedy administration that public schools have a shortage of 600,000 teachers." I also received two letters: one agreeing with and one protesting what I presumably had said.

Undoubtedly, the memory of the difference between "teachers" and "teaching" affected the way I framed questions when, some six years later, I examined policy issues around the presumed physician shortage. There, too, professionals stated there was a large shortage often estimated at some 40,000 physicians. When I once asked a high official of the National Institutes of Health where that figure came from, I was told, "Whatever we have, we are 40,000 short." That answer also piqued my interest. The "teacher shortage" incidence did teach me an important lesson: when examining the physician shortage I didn't leave it to a snappy sentence as in "there's no shortage of doctors only a shortage of doctoring!" I invited the reader to focus on "physicians' services" rather than physicians, arguing that the role that physician assistants, nurse practitioners, public health nurses, and pharmacists played and could play affected the number of physicians the nation would need. The argument that we needed to examine what physicians do and what skills are needed to do the various tasks was well-received. Perhaps, however, that was because, having learned a lesson, I presented my ideas in far more than a very few brief sentences.

The lesson that one shouldn't assume that everyone is on the same wave length and, therefore, that everyone will fill in the missing links in the argument the same way was clear. Terseness may not be a virtue. Not everyone thinks like an economist or sociologist or political scientist or expresses ideas in quite the same way. Thus, while it is important that each practitioner of a discipline be precise, it is also important to expand on the thought process that leads from A to B and then to C. Failing that, one may end up on the front page of the *Times*.

Context Matters

Of course, the failure to amplify the thought pattern involved in the choice of words is only one of the problems that can arise in the selection of the language to be used in conveying information to individuals who have not been trained in the policy adviser's particular discipline and in its language and thought patterns. Sometimes the words one uses change with the perspective of the speaker. Indeed, even the same speaker describing the same event, but doing so at different times and conditions, may inadvertently or purposively select words that alter and sometimes are designed to alter the way the message is received. One incident captures that condition.

I joined the faculty of the University of North Carolina (Chapel Hill) in the fall of 1952. As a consequence of the salary negotiation process, Carolina's initial offer of $4,000 for a twelve month year (with one month vacation) had been increased to $4,100. Some years later I was told that I was a bad bargainer: the university had been prepared to go all the way to $4,200. A pity I didn't hold out a bit longer since an extra $100 would have been quite helpful.

One year later, in October of 1953, I met the dean of the School of Business Administration of which the Department of Economics was a part as he was walking up the stairs to the coffee lounge and I was going down. He stopped me and asked whether I was enjoying the "merit increase" I had been granted: "How do you like your 3.5 percent increase? I recognize it may not have seemed so much, but I'm sure you are finding the $144 a year, $12 a month very helpful." I told him that perhaps he was mistaken about the change in salary since I had not seen any increase in my pay check. He was surprised since the adjustment was to have been effective July 1 and this was October. While agreeing that I'd surely have noticed the increase, he suggested I might want to double check and told me that he would do so as well by calling the financial office to determine what had happened.

The next day I was asked to come to his office. I remember his statement: "The financial office made some kind of an error and didn't enter my recommendation on its books. They can rectify the matter, but are unable to do so retroactively. Your pay for the remaining months will increase, but there is no way to give you the $12 a month you should have received these past four months. I'm really sorry that's the case, but after all it's not so bad: the loss, after all, is only $12 a month." As the dispenser of "largesse," he felt the increase of 3.5 percent was something to be noticed and appreciated. As the person who couldn't make it retroactive, he concluded the loss was of little meaning or consequence: "only $12 a month, hardly to be missed."

Consider how—in policy debates as well as in more casual conversations—the same words (or as in this case, numbers) may have different meanings, depending on where one sits. The words we choose sometimes can confuse. The policy adviser must be precise lest she or he be misunderstood. Thus, for example, we all (though, as we shall see, not quite all) decry the "high and rapidly rising costs of medical care." One might wonder how it can be that year after year state and federal officials, columnists and editorial writers, employers, insurance companies, the general public decry the increases and, yet, no effective and long lasting constraints have been put in place. What few "success stories" have occurred have been effective in limited venues or geographic areas and sometimes for relatively brief periods of time—perhaps a placebo or Hawthorne effect that "works" simply because something new is being tried—and then "costs" have reverted to their "normal" upward trend line. Often, cost-containment efforts can be described as processes in which programs are instituted, stay in place for a period of time, are dismantled and are replaced by yet other "new initiatives." How does one explain the failure to act on a matter that almost everyone agrees is of such importance? One hypothesis is that, though increases in health care costs are deplored, the measures that might control such increases would have additional and negative consequences. It is as if the medicine to be administered would cure the disease but the various side effects would be equally or perhaps even more distressing.

There is a second hypothesis. Perhaps some who decry the rapid and inexorable increase in costs are fearful that cost-control measures would reduce the availability of care and that that burden would fall on them rather than on the total population. Surely one can understand that under those circumstances they would oppose such measures. Such behavior might be especially true among population groups that use more medical care—e.g., the disabled and, perhaps, the elderly—or feel powerless to protect their rights—as, for example members of minority groups or persons who are poor.

There is an additional, a third hypothesis. We may well be correct in believing that many of us decry the increase in health care costs, but are incorrect when we behave as if "many" means "all." Perhaps it is the case that arrayed against those who would slow down the rate of growth are others who are not at all troubled, perhaps even pleased, with the high level of what we call "costs" and the inexorable increases and are prepared to oppose cost containment programs. That this is not an unreasonable hypothesis is made clear by an examination of one's perspective and language. Economists remind us that one person's—say, the patient's—costs are another person's—say, the physician's—income, a point that seems obvious after it is raised, but whose implications are overlooked until it is pointed out. Of course it is true that there are many more patients and potential patients than there are providers of care, many more persons who would prefer lower costs than persons, institutions, and organizations that would prefer higher costs, many more patient payers than provider payees. Yet there is a body of literature in political science that takes note of the fact that intensity of feeling on the part of a few about an issue that has a large effect on them may be far more significant than the diffused interests of the many for whom the issue, though important, is only one of many matters of concern. That is what makes possible the influence of "special interests" and the growth and power of lobbyists. Whether one sees the increase in costs by payers as something to be deplored or the growth in income to payees as something to be praised, albeit privately, depends upon where one sits and, perforce, the language that one might use.

Nor, for that matter, is that the only problem with the word "costs" or the phrase "costs of medical care." As used, these words are extraordinarily imprecise and neither define "costs" or tell us very much about possible actions that might control them. Just before writing these words I attended a luncheon talk by the former governor of Massachusetts, Michael Dukakis, in which he addressed the high costs of medical care and reminded the audience that there had been a time when a regulatory mechanism was in place in Massachusetts as well as in many other states that called for health planning at the state level and in intrastate regions, certificate-of-need approval for new capital investment, and effective rate control on payments or reimbursements to hospitals and nursing facilities. He argued that it was time to return to such regulatory mechanisms. Thus, he was advocating measures that would affect capacity and prices. In the discussion period that followed it became clear that some in the audience were not especially interested in the price issue and did not believe that prices had very much to do with what they considered to be the "cost" problem. Their concern was with expenditures, the product of price times quantity. They argued that costs were high—they meant dollar outlays not prices—because of the number of interventions by physicians, the number of visits, and the number of procedures. In their view, the payoff on the cost front would come as a consequence of learning how to control volume, that is, quantity. It is not clear where they stood on measures to affect capacity, but it was quite clear that they were not especially concerned about prices. Yet, all those who spoke—whether they were speaking about prices or expenditures—used the same word: "costs" as in "costs of health care."

There is little confusion if I say that the cost of coffee has gone up. Everyone knows I must be referring to the price per pound or per cup across the counter. So it is with a whole variety of goods and services. Similarly, there is little confusion if I state that the cost of police protection has increased. That quite correctly conjures up an image of an increase in the budget for police. While an increase in the price per pound for coffee may lead to my spending more

money on coffee, it may not do so. That depends on what economists call "the elasticity of demand," the degree to which I reduce
consumption because of the price increase. When I write that there
has been an increase in the cost of coffee the reader knows I am
writing about price not expenditure. Similarly, while an increase in
the cost of police protection may derive from an increase in salaries
of individual police officers, the reader knows that when I write
of an increase in costs of police protection I am writing about an
increase in how much we spend, about an increase in outlays. But
what do I mean when I state that costs of medical care are increasing? Do I mean that the price for an office visit, x-ray, or day in
the hospital went up or do I mean that we are spending more in
total for/on these and other units of service? Am I speaking about
prices or expenditures?

The price level and the rate of price inflation are measured by and
are of considerable interest to the Bureau of Labor Statistics (BLS)
in the Department of Labor. If, on the other hand, we are spending
more the matter is of great interest to those who deal with budgets.
They must ascertain whether this is due to an increase in prices or
in volume since the policy actions called for would vary with their
diagnosis. Controlling prices is a very different matter than controlling volume. Indeed, one can conceive of policies that would help
on one front, but do harm on the other.

A long time ago a group of fellows in the Center for Community
Health and Medical Care at Harvard Medical School and I played
a game called "If you were the president." One participant was
designated as the president of the United States. I note that already
almost forty years ago our group had a woman "president." Her
advisers raised concerns about the costs of medical care and called
upon departments in the executive branch—as represented by other
fellows—to consider what actions would be appropriate and effective if we were to contain the increase in costs. The "game" had
many facets, but the first task always had to be to define "cost."

We discovered that the actions the president would take depended
on the definition of costs that was accepted. Thus, for example, if
the president listened to the Office of Management and Budget
(OMB) as it said "we have to reduce costs [expenditures] for medi-

cal care," she might call for programs designed to reduce length of stay in hospitals, thus reducing hospital expenditures. Yet, what if the Bureau of Labor Statistics responded: "But that means that the least sick will leave the hospital and the most sick would remain and on average the patient in the hospital bed would be sicker than before the policy had been implemented. In turn that means that the hospital day for the now sicker average patient would cost more and that inflation, as measured by the consumer price index, would increase. The public will not know that expenditures went down, but will be well aware and troubled that prices went up."

Conversely, suppose that the BLS came to the president and stated that inflationary pressures were mounting and the Federal Reserve might be forced to increase interest rates and, therefore, that the president needed to intervene in order to restrain inflation. In order to restrain hospital price inflation the president might consider suggesting that healthy people who wouldn't require intensive or extensive nursing care or hi-tech hospital services fill all empty hospital beds, thus reducing the average daily hospital charge. But what would a "fill the beds" policy do to total expenditures, the budget, and the comfort level at the Office of Management and Budget? Thus, the actions to be taken depended critically on the definition of costs: is the president concerned about inflation in prices or increases in expenditure?

Of course, all that is hypothetical. What is not at all hypothetical is that the seeds of confusion both about analysis and about policy are sown if we use the word "cost" to mean different things and aren't at all clear of what we speak. Words are precious. Confusion in language and in analysis cannot but help lead to confusion in understanding and in policy.

Physicians and Social Scientists: A Contrast

I have referred to the difficulty that may ensue—as, for example, in the use of such words as "producer," "consumer," and "patient compliance"—when words mean something different to persons with different backgrounds. The problem in communication may also arise because persons in different disciplines not only think about different problems, but do so in different ways. Thus, for example, the economist who is advising the decision maker who is a physician must recognize that how economists think is not how doctors think. I am not referring to neurons, the right side and left side of our brains, or to innate characteristics, although I recognize that perhaps those lead to self-selection into different disciplines or subject areas of interest. I refer instead to the perspective that is brought even to the same field of inquiry. One can see this in the ways that social scientists and physicians view a similar problem and hear the same word. That the policy adviser must recognize this difference is self-evident.

Social scientists (certainly economists) seek to generalize. That's how we measure things; that's how we think. Speak to an economist about poverty and it is likely that she or he will cite the dimension of the problem: how many persons and families are poor, what recent trends have been and how those trends compare with the past, perhaps even what factors seem to be associated with poverty. Conversely, speak to a physician about poverty and it is likely that she or he will remember Mrs. Jones who was seen just last week and who confided that in an effort to save money she had been skipping some of her medications—as in, "I take my blood pressure pills only when I'm not feeling well"—and to whom the physician gave some of the samples the pharmaceutical representative had left. The social scientist thinks of the general phenomenon; the physician thinks of the particular patient. The economist thinks of poverty and may never have met a poor person; the physician thinks of the poor person and has not considered the phenomenon called "poverty." I can testify that service on committees that included members of the medical community as well as social scientists representing different disciplines—each person with his or her singular background and experience—has often required learning how to communicate and understand each other's language and thought processes.

In part, I exaggerate the chasm. Conditions are improving. As an increasing proportion of social scientists move into applied areas of research and participate in research that involves field work and gathering rather than simply using data, more and more investigators encounter flesh-and-blood individuals and gain respect for institutions and institutional arrangements and constraints, for the strengths and, as well, the limitations on the applicability of theory. They become aware of the importance of ethnic, geographic, cultural, social, and economic differences between groups and become more cognizant of the need to focus increased attention on what might be termed micro aspects of the human conditions. They learn to understand the language and perspective of other disciplines. In similar fashion, an increasing number of medical students, residents, and practicing and research physicians have become more knowledgeable about epidemiology and biostatistics as well as the social sciences and exhibit an increasing interest in moving away from the bedside of the patient as their primary or only locus of interest and activity and examining group phenomena. Nevertheless, differences do remain.

It was those differences that impressed themselves upon me when—in my first experience in a medical school—I began teaching a course on the organization and financing of medical care to first and second year medical students at Harvard Medical School some forty years ago (a time when both financing and organization of medical care were much, much simpler). I realized that other than my course the rest of the medical school curriculum focused student attention on the patient (and often on an even smaller unit, an organ or, ignoring the patient, on a disease). Conversely, my lectures on infant mortality and its socio-economic context, health insurance, prepaid group practice, and similar topics dealt with very different issues involving groups of people and fell into a category of studies that these prospective physicians had hoped to leave behind in their transition from undergraduate to medical school days. I wanted them to think of people; they wanted to think of the person. I wanted to focus on society and to some degree on dollars; they wanted to focus on the patient in need. I was aware that in a real sense I was fighting a losing battle: they wanted to become doctors, saw themselves as treating patients, and believed that that is what the great physicians on the faculty were about. All of the pressures within the school and from "society" were focused on their interaction with the patient who had a problem and who needed help.

It was as if they had been taken into a forest and handed an ax, told to fell a tree and thin the grove and I had intervened to tell them that they really ought to learn the principles of mechanics so they could hold the ax "correctly" and, as well, listen to a lecture on ecology and consider the implications of what they were about to do: how trees grew and why and when groves needed thinning, and so forth. The pressure was to buy into the "either-or" concept that held that either one was a good—in the Harvard expectation, a superb—clinician or researcher or one was knowledgeable about health care delivery and its social and economic dimensions. Presumably one couldn't learn both: either one would know how to deal with the medical problems of the Medicare eligible patient or one would know how Medicare came into being and what it covered.

I was very critical of the emphasis—what I felt was overemphasis—devoted to issues "at the bedside of the patient." And that was aside from my view that ambulatory care was being "shortchanged" since students spent most of their clinical time in the hospital and literally at the bedside of the patient while most often those who are ill are not hospitalized and encounter their physician in an office setting. My problem was that treating one patient at a time would not address the general problem of asthma, of lead paint, or of infant mortality. I was interested in policy, wanted to further change in the economics of health care (broadly defined), knew that changes would have to involve the medical community, that physicians would influence the direction and pace of change, and, therefore, that physicians needed to know more about those areas. My problem was that participation in health care policy discussions required a knowledge base that many, if not most, students as well as practicing physicians found far less exciting and important than the presumed alternative: the acquisition of clinical knowledge. To me the issue seemed to be how we would communicate across those intellectual gulfs.

And then one day I had an epiphany. I imagined that I was lying in a hospital bed and that one of my former students, by now a practicing and perhaps renowned physician, came into the room and greeted me: "Hi, Professor Fein [at the time in the "olden" days of 1968, even students, let alone bank tellers and salespersons whom one had never met and might never meet again, had not yet developed the habit of greeting everyone by first name] remember me? I'm so-and-so. Surely, you remember me; you gave me an A in that course that talked about health and society. It's really good to see you, though I'm sorry that it's under such conditions. Well, let me tell you about your medical problem. You'll be pleased to know that we can take care of it. Still, I know that when I tell you about the various other things we could do with the resources required to treat you, for example, how much we might reduce unwanted pregnancies or increase smoking cessation programs, you'll agree that we should devote our efforts to those problems. No reflection on you, but dealing with any one of them would have a far greater positive societal impact. As you can tell, I really learned a lot in your course."

As I thought about and was not particularly thrilled by that presumed encounter, I, the imaginary patient, developed a new respect for all that the clinical faculty was doing to prepare our students to take care of patients. I realized—and felt relieved—that the rest of the medical school faculty was working to assure that the imagined scenario would not play out. I still believed in what I was teaching and in its importance, ·but the school's priorities also seemed to make sense. Some attention needed to be paid to what might broadly be called "social medicine,"—population health problems are not solved through one-on-one acute care interventions and physicians need to understand what Medicare covers and what social forces led to its enactment—but the role of the physician is not the same role as that of the economist or of the allocator of society's resources or of the adviser who helps those who determines community health care priorities. Economists are not physicians and physicians are not economists. Nor should they be. Since physicians are professionals and persons who historically have had and will continue to have considerable input into medical and health care policy, it behooves them to understand far more than the technical aspects of medicine. Nevertheless, I was quite certain that when I would be ill I would want treatment, not a lecture on Blue Cross and its strengths and weaknesses.

Of course, that did not mean total neglect of the language of the epidemiologist, the issues involving health care disparities, the social context of disease, and the problems that patients have with insurance coverage, with access, and with economic and social barriers to care. These were additional matters that physicians needed to be familiar with in order to help patients and to participate in policy discussions. Undoubtedly, many diagnoses can be made without that "extra" knowledge, but treating the patient most often requires that one know and understand the patient and the world he or she inhabits. There is a role, therefore, for both kinds of knowledge: I was glad my former student earned an "A" in my course and I was more than pleased that his experience at Harvard Medical School would not lead him to lecture patients about preferred alternative uses for the resources required to treat their ailments.

This story might strike some as being about an ancient time in medical education and, in any event, of little relevance to the policy process. It is true that there is far more attention paid in today's curriculum to epidemiology, disease prevention and health promotion, health disparities, and issues relevant to global health. More medical students take courses and/or receive joint degrees in schools of public health, government and public policy, business, law, and in the social sciences—though, in many cases they become administrators or consultants and leave the practice of medicine. Nevertheless, the issue raised in the imaginary conversation between me, the hospitalized patient, and my physician remains important. It reminds us of the power that physicians have and that, appropriately, derives from their expert knowledge. We need to be aware that power—as, for example, in allocating scarce resources—might be exercised inappropriately, that is, beyond the physician's area of individual responsibility and expertise. It should also remind us that the problem I raise—the difference in thought pattern and, therefore, in the use of words and choice of language, between the social scientist and the physician—is part of a more general problem that often arises in discourse between the generalist and the practitioner in an applied area. It is a problem often encountered by policy advisers and analysts as they pursue their craft and is resolved in the same manner as many problems we have discussed are resolved: by a search for balance.

There's Rationing and There's Rationing

I have raised the allocation issue and suggested that since the physician's responsibility is to the patient whom he is treating, he is not the appropriate person to determine whether the individual patient's care represents an optimal use of available resources. The patient believes and should believe that the physician's responsibility is to the patient—not to the HMO, the insurance company, or even to "society." Completeness requires that I note that some would offer a much simpler answer to the allocation question. They might argue that I shouldn't worry that courses in social medicine and social responsibility will "contaminate" the student and leave the future physician in a schizophrenic state torn between his duty to the patient and his responsibility to society. They would suggest that my attempt to seek "balance" is misplaced and would argue that the marketplace, not the physician, should determine the allocation of scarce resources. Language, consensus, communication, and negotiation become less important; the market and my ability or inability to pay for the charges incurred for the care ought to determine the end of the story. If I choose to pay and can do so, I should receive care; if I cannot, I should do without. In their view, my former student should not interfere with the presumably free market.

They would criticize me for raising the specter of "rationing," a word that they would use to describe the situation in which my physician denied me care in favor of someone else or of some other activity using medical resources. On the face of it, those "free marketers" and I are in agreement in questioning whether the individual physician—even had he or she had a dozen courses in social responsibility—should be making rationing decisions in the context of his or her intersection with an individual patient. But there we part company, for the source of my difficulty is not the concept of rationing but the locus of allocative decision making. For me the critical issue is not the word "rationing," but the mechanism by which rationing decisions are reached. Since policy debates in the health field, most especially as they relate to universal health insurance, often revolve around issues that are perceived as leading to or calling for the presumably new phenomenon, "rationing," the different perceptions of the meanings and issues invoked by the extraordinarily powerful word "rationing"—a word whose use has helped derail various legislative initiatives—bear examination.

Though many choose to overlook it or to define it in terms less charged than "rationing," in today's United States access to medical care is already rationed. The rationing mechanism relies on price: those who have health insurance or sufficient monetary resources do move to the front of the line and do receive more care. Since "rationing" is a "bad" word we may choose not to use the term "rationing" or "price rationing" to describe the situation that precludes individuals from purchasing various goods and services including health insurance and health care. Nevertheless, that is an accurate descriptor: the price system determines the allocation, that is, rations, all sorts of things including medical services. If care were to be allocated, apportioned, or "rationed" on a basis other than by income and price we would need some other mechanism to determine those allocations. One possibility, of course, is that the matter is left in the hands and to the decision of individual physicians while we make believe that the sum of all those individual decisions would represent the collective judgment of society. That mechanism has one important virtue: the criteria for rationing are not made explicit and do not require our participation or ratification. Just as the "invisible hand" of the market insulates us from a feeling of responsibility—the impersonal market, not you or I determines who receives and who does without—so, too, with the quiet and non-transparent physician decisions. We can sleep soundly; we are not responsible for denying care.

Nevertheless, whatever the benefits that some may ascribe to rationing decisions that are not made explicit and that are made without the patient and family knowing what might have been, surely these presumed advantages are outweighed by the ad hoc nature of decisions made by individual physicians, each with his or her own standards and value system, determining who shall and who shall not be treated and how. If rationing is required, the choice of technologies and procedures that should be available and under what circumstances ought to be a societal decision made by those designated to do so at a societal level. I do not suggest that each of us would necessarily agree with the rationing decisions implied by those societal decisions, but surely they would be less arbitrary and could be much more transparent than those made by individual physicians. It is no accident that there is increasing questioning of physician decisions about such allocation issues, as in "end-of-life" situations.

Furthermore, most of us in fact do not find price rationing a particularly desirable allocation mechanism. A majority of legislators and of the general population is willing to interfere with the market distribution of health resources—as, for example, in requiring that emergency rooms treat all who come through their doors regardless of income or insurance status—and supports calls for even more interference. The wide variety of social programs mounted by various levels of government as well as by voluntary not-for-profit social agencies provides ample evidence that Americans are uncomfortable with the market as the ultimate distributive device. Subsidized housing, food banks, free medical care, and fuel assistance are only a few of the arenas in which we have "interfered" with the market and have quite consciously and deliberately chosen a different mode of rationing.

Many nations have turned away from the market when they have sought fairer and more equitable distribution of a particular good or service. That is true as well for the United States. When our nation faced a meat shortage—an imbalance between the supply of meat offered and the demand for meat at the prevailing Office of Price Administration controlled price—during World War II, it adopted a system of non-price rationing. It did not simply permit meat prices to increase in order to contract or stifle demand and, thus, "eliminate," that is, define away, the shortage. Nor did it give individual butchers the authority to increase the allocation to Mrs. Jones and reduce it to Mr. Smith as they saw fit. Rather we distributed ration stamps on the basis of demographic characteristics designed to achieve "fairness." These stamps or coupons, together with monetary payments, were required for meat purchase. We chose to distribute the available supply of meat on a basis that we considered equitable, rather than on the basis of market allocation.

It is possible that it takes a crisis to force us to resort to that approach. Most often, after all, we expect prices to bring supply and demand into balance and, by definition, eliminate potential shortages. In 1967 the *New York Times* headlined a story that it reported from Poland, "Poland Raises Meat Prices 16.7% to Ease Shortage; Displeasure Is Shown."[7] Yet the article stated that "Polish sources stressed that no major improvement in meat supplies could be expected in the next few years." The amount of meat per person would not increase, but—*mirabile dictu*—the shortage would be "eased." In that context, the "shortage" had little to do with need, desire, or supply. Rather the shortage was eliminated by raising the price and thus rationing some who would have tried to purchase meat at lower prices out of the market because they could not afford the higher price. Ergo, the shortage—which has nothing to do with how much meat Poles had, but with an imbalance between supply and demand—no longer existed. The shortage was eliminated by reducing demand and thus eliminating the imbalance, by the invisible hand. Presumably Poland had not had to resort to the blunt instrument called "rationing."

Consider how different a World War II radio show on rationing presented the same issue. That broadcast illustrates the point and also makes clear that one's reaction to rationing depends on context, on how the matter is presented, that is whether it involves some collective enterprise or appears arbitrary.

> *Radio Announcer:* Americans are experiencing the horrors of rationing.
>
> *Woman:* Now we are going to have a new system of rationing, I hear.
>
> *Grocer:* Yup, that's right. Going to start point rationing pretty soon, they tell me.
>
> *Woman:* Why on earth do they have to do that? We have a perfectly simple system for sugar and coffee. I can't make heads or tails of it. I wish someone would explain to me why we're going from one thing to another.

Announcer: How many of us have heard just that sort of conversation during the past few days since the announcement by the Secretary of Agriculture Wickard that canned, dried and frozen fruits and vegetables would be rationed within a short time. Well, we have someone here who is prepared to answer some questions that have arisen and explain what these new developments are all about, Mr. Paul O'Leary, Deputy Administrator in Charge of Rationing in the Office of Price Administration.

Mr. O'Leary: Good evening.

Announcer: Mr. O'Leary, I think you're the right man to answer questions that seem to be bothering Mrs. Hendricks and her grocer. They're here right now.

Mr. O'Leary: I'd be glad to try. Tell me, Mrs. Hendricks, why do you particularly want canned tomatoes rather than some fresh vegetables?

Woman: Well, Mr. O'Leary, it's so hard to plan my husband's meals. He very often works overtime and doesn't get home to dinner at all. I'd like to have a canned vegetable on hand. Fresh vegetables do spoil, and I don't know just when I will have time to use them.

Mr. O'Leary: That partly answers one of your questions about the why of this canned food rationing, doesn't it, Mrs. Hendricks? The Army has to plan meals for over a million American soldiers scattered all over the earth and they have to be fed canned foods because only canned foods will be useful for months. Imagine what fresh tomatoes would look like when they got to North Africa.

Grocer: Hey, that's right Mrs. Hendricks, I know what spoilage means with fresh fruits and vegetables. Are we feeding soldiers a great amount of canned goods overseas, Mr. O'Leary?

Mr. O'Leary: Yes, indeed, we certainly are! For the Army and Navy, and our fighting allies as well. They're fighting on our side, and they can do a better job with some good substantial American food under their belts.

Grocer: Well, Mr. O'Leary, that's going to take an awful lot of canned stuff.

Mr. O'Leary: Yup, we've got a lot. We're at peak production as far as food is concerned.

Woman: Then I still don't see why we need rationing.

Mr. O'Leary: Even with that super production of ours, we are still going to have to cut down our consumption of canned food.

Grocer: Mr. O'Leary, you mean rationing?

Mr. O'Leary: That's right. We've got to divide among our civilian population what we have left after feeding our fighting men. And that means there'll be *a little less for some of us, but a fair share for all of us* [my emphasis].

Woman: Well, I'm all in favor of seeing those boys get first chance of whatever there is.

Grocer: Mrs. Hendricks has a son in the army herself, Mr. O'Leary.[8]

On my CD of sounds of the Second World War this segment ends with a song "…Oh, there may be a shortage of sugar, of aluminum pots and such. But there won't be a shortage of love when we love each other so much…" The lyricist fortunately recognized the difference between love and sugar, aluminum pots, and such and concluded that love did not have to be rationed.

We should take notice of the key phrase in Mr. O'Leary's response "a little less for some of us, but a fair share for all," a phrase that was easier to say and an implied program that was easier to implement during a war that was supported by the vast majority of Americans and in which we were all called upon to contribute to a collective effort, to sacrifice and share.

My dictionary states that ration "implies apportionment and, often equal sharing…it is freely extended to scarce things made available equally or equitably in accord with need." Rationing, in turn, means "to distribute equitably." Neither price rationing nor arbitrary decisions by individual physicians, grocers, oil distributors, and so forth meet that definition. The "equitable" perspective is summarized in a short essay that the dean of social administration and social welfare, Richard Titmuss, wrote shortly before his death in 1973. The last paragraph in the essay describing his experience at the National Health Service as a cancer patient reads: "Among all the other experiences I had, another which stands out is that of a young West Indian from Trinidad, aged 25, with cancer of the rectum. His appointment was the same as mine for radium treatment—ten o'clock every day. Sometimes he went into the Theratron Room first; sometimes I did. What determined waiting was quite simply the vagaries of London traffic—not race, religion, colour or class."[9]

The physician and the policy maker have different roles to play. The problem of reconciling care for the individual and care for the community will not disappear. Physicians are not likely to become economists and economists, surely, will not become physicians. And that is how it should be. It would not hurt if more physicians knew more about "social medicine" and population issues. It would also not hurt if more economists knew more about the every day issues in practicing medicine, in staffing an emergency room and triaging patients, in operating an institution called a hospital that is part medical facility and part hotel. Indeed, it is more likely that physicians will acquire the suggested breadth of knowledge than that economists and other social scientists will. The former, as noted, have opportunity to take a variety of formal and informal courses specifically designed to expose the physician to the perspective of other disciplines. The obverse does not hold: medical schools do not typically offer mini-courses deigned to add to the social scientist's understanding of the world of medicine: how physicians think and what they think about.

We do think differently and we think about different things. We use the same words, but react differently to them. On one occasion when I came into my physician's office he seemed especially joyful, greeting me with an exclamation that he had looked forward to this visit since it provided him with an opportunity to talk about the problems of the health care system and where it was heading. It was not clear why the prospects of such a conversation would make him joyful, but in any case I tried to beg off with a statement that I was tired of that discussion, that that's what I talk about for a living, and that there must be some other topic that might engage us, as for example, my health or how the Red Sox might do. He expressed his disappointment, told me that he had looked forward to the conversation all day, but understood where I was coming from. Though my behavior was unfair, he would respect my wishes.

Nevertheless, by way of explanation for his choice of topic, he insisted on telling me that when, some many decades earlier, he first set up practice after various residencies and fellowships, he and a number of his friends opened their offices in Boston/Brookline/ Newton. They and their wives would get together for dinner once a month. He stated that invariably the wives complained because "in those early years all we would talk about was medicine." He then told me, "They still complain, but now it's about the fact that today all we talk about is economics." By "economics" he surely meant the conditions of practice, the paper work, the intersection with multiple insurance companies and an even larger number of different insurance policies each with its own structure of covered benefits, and the ever present regulatory and administrative pressures. I could not help but feel for him. I tried to cheer him up by taking some license and noting that when I was a young economist, a group of us and our wives would go to dinner and our wives complained because "all we talked about was economics." I added that as the years passed and we became older the wives still complained, "But today the complaints are because all we talk about now is medicine!" Of course, just as his "economics" meant the economics of his practice, so by "medicine" I meant my state of health. Both of us know more about the "other's" world, but our perspectives and how we think about that other world remain and will remain quite different.

The policy adviser is required to understand that his or her advice will be heard and read by many persons, each with a particular and necessarily limited knowledge base, set of experiences, and perspective. Each, therefore, may read the policy memorandum differently. The policy adviser must anticipate this phenomenon. Nevertheless, while important, it is not enough to couch recommendations in a language that one hopes maximizes commonality and minimizes misunderstanding. Consider the answer that two members of the President's Council of Economic Advisers gave at the end of their first year in office when a business and economics reporter asked what they felt constituted their most important first year accomplishment. Independently they responded "The education of a President." The policy adviser who anticipates a continuing relationship with his or her principal—or long term service on a policy committee with a stable membership—will find it useful to invest the time and effort to "educate" his and her colleagues and, in turn, to be educated about their words, thoughts, ideas, and agendas.

Words make a difference. Words have an impact. The policy adviser must treat them with care and the respect due a precious commodity.

3

Defining the Policy Options and Issues

The initial task of the policy adviser and of her or his principal is to define the objective of any new policy. Only when that has been done can one examine the different ways to attain the goal one seeks, the various benefits yielded by the options, and the time required both to begin to make a visible difference and to claim success. Sometimes a set of policies has a favorable impact, but the results, though worth pursuing, are long in coming. If that is the case one may support those meritorious policies, but—in an effort to maintain public backing for change—also actively favor efforts that would yield more rapid or visible advances towards the goal. The choice of options is never easy, but it becomes even more difficult when one recognizes that few policies are one dimensional. Most create multiple results, some positive, others negative, along a wide spectrum with results that cannot easily be compared.

The matter of multiple ways to attain a goal and multiple kinds of benefits from various actions was brought home to me almost half a century ago during the John F. Kennedy presidency. One of the administration's central economic objectives was to increase the United States rate of economic growth. In part, this emphasis stemmed from the need to eliminate the "missile gap." Presumably the Russians had more missiles than we and expansion of our capability could be accomplished more readily and with less impact on other domestic and international programs only if our economy grew more rapidly. As we discovered later, there was no gap and in any event both the U.S. and the USSR had more than enough atomic weaponry and missile delivery systems to destroy each other. Thus the need to fill the "gap," even had one existed, was not all that compelling, unless one believed that as the world was being destroyed the side with the most missiles left would be able to claim some sort of victory.

But the rationale for more rapid economic growth did not rest solely on the missile gap. It was argued that in the context of the Cold War between the USA and the USSR, we needed to grow rapidly because, given relative and projected rates of growth of the two adversaries, some decades hence Soviet Gross National Product would overtake ours. In order to stay ahead we had to grow more rapidly.

All of us are familiar with such projections in various fields of activity. In regard to national health expenditures, for example, the following question is often posed: when, given current trends in which health expenditures increase at a faster rate than does the Gross Domestic Product and, therefore, absorb an ever greater share of the GDP, will health care consume the entire GDP? Such projections can convert even the most skeptical economist into one who believes that market forces will bring things into some sort of balance. We can rest assured that national health expenditures will never absorb the nation's entire product. This is a case where one can violate the "never say never" injunction.

Whatever the international rationale for the concern with increasing economic growth, the case for expansion did not need to rest on competition with the Soviet Union. That rational seemed most important in the 1960s Cold War era and especially since we seemed to find ourselves in what clearly would be a prolonged, protracted, and perhaps never-ending struggle with a formidable adversary. Nevertheless, even if those imperatives may have been irrelevant both because there was no gap and because early 1960 trends in the USSR would not be sustained, everyone was aware that accelerated and sustained economic growth would help meet "domestic needs." Growth could add to disposable income and provide additional resources for individuals to raise their standard of living; growth could provide additional revenues to local, state, and federal coffers and make it possible to expand expenditures for the various activities of government such as education, health care, transportation, infrastructure, and defense; growth would make possible a reduction in tax rates even while maintaining or increasing total tax revenues.

Given the emphasis on economic growth, the Council of Economic Advisers devoted a full chapter of its 1962 Economic Report to that issue.[1] Believing that growth could be stimulated by appropriate interventions even beyond traditional actions advocated in relation to fiscal and monetary policy, the report advanced a number of policy proposals designed to help create the necessary conditions for expansion in different sectors of the economy. Among the items listed as basic determinants of a society's productive capacity in any given year were: "The number of people available for employment, the number of hours they wish to work, their incentives and motivations, and their health, general education, occupational desires, and vocational skills." Thus, the Council argued that we needed more investment in human resources. Bob Lampman, long-time student of the American income distribution and of social expenditures, and I wrote sections on the contributions that more and deeper education, better health, and the elimination of racial discrimination would make to economic growth. We suggested policies that were desirable in their own right and that at the same time would contribute to growth.

The report was transmitted to Congress on January 20, 1962. This was followed by hearings before the Joint Economic Committee whose members interrogated the Council members. We knew whether a question would be friendly or hostile by the opening words addressed to the chairman of the CEA: "Professor Heller" meant we were in trouble; "Dr. Heller" meant we stood a chance; "Mr. Heller" meant we were in friendly territory. Some of the questions, as for example, when Senator Jacob Javits of New York inquired how much racial discrimination was costing the economy, were answered with a more-or-less standard response: "My staff will provide an answer within ten days and submit it for the record."

Subsequently, months after things had settled down, a number of us had an opportunity to discuss several of the matters raised in the report with a distinguished visiting European economist. When we explained the basis for our views about the importance of education as an economic ingredient that would help stimulate economic growth by raising productivity, he responded with a note of skepticism. It was not that higher levels of education would not be beneficial, but he thought that relative to other possible policies we most probably overemphasized the matter. He noted that a much larger proportion of students attended college in the United States than in his nation and, further, that an extraordinarily high proportion of our students took a course in economics and did so from the superb text by Paul Samuelson. Thus, a much higher proportion of Americans had an exposure to Samuelson and a greater understanding of formal economics was embodied in their human capital than was the case at home. Presumably that created conditions that helped improve our economic performance: more Americans understood (at least in an analytic sense) the utility of appropriate monetary and fiscal policies. Yet his nation, with less emphasis on education, had a higher rate of economic growth than that of the United States. He suggested that the explanation for this phenomenon was not really complex: Scandinavian nations pursued specific full-employment policies, including manpower policies and worker training and retraining, while the U.S., though aware of the need for such policies had not adopted them with any vigorous effort and was languishing with over 6 percent unemployment.

He did not negate the importance of education, but its contribution to economic growth, though positive, was dominated by full employment's contribution to growth. He could have added that the beneficial impacts of improvement in health, education, and of the elimination of racial discrimination even if important, would take a considerable time in coming.

The lesson embodied in that anecdote applies to all sorts of matters in the public policy arena. Of course, the case for certain policies need not rest on the important, but limited goal of raising the GDP. More education, better health, and the elimination of discrimination are worthy social goals whether their economic impact is large or marginal. Nevertheless, while not discounting the significance of even marginal economic advances—and in such fields as health, education, and investment in human capital the margin can be quite wide—our Scandinavian colleague's comments served as a reminder that it is also important to try to move things in big ways.

Thus, for example, I could imagine that today our visiting economist might say, "I see you Americans are concerned about racial disparities in health and health care and that considerable sums are being expended by all levels of government and foundations to study ways to reduce those disparities. That's fine, but I believe that your failure to deal with the inequality in your income distribution and with the large number of adults and children who live in poverty will mean that you will not really be able to come to grips with those disparities. You can improve things at the margin and I certainly believe that is worth doing, but system failures are repaired by system change, not by operating at the margin. Implicit in that, of course, is the observation that to change the way systems perform you must understand why they perform the way they do."

The issue, once again, is one of balance. We can and should operate at both the micro and the macro level. Unfortunately, that does not always occur. Since system change often is more difficult to accomplish and is far riskier than incremental change, it is easy to understand that those who advance policy options may be biased in favor of the incremental. It is necessary to be sensitive to the problem and to encourage policy advisers to break out of the self-imposed boundaries that limit their analysis and constrain policy development and implementation and to "think big." Marginal changes may yield marginal results. The frustration and disappointments that may follow may lead to a conviction that "nothing works," thus making it ever more difficult to undertake even limited marginal actions.

Should Politics Affect Policy?

Among the first thing that an adviser or a committee of advisers must do when a principal requests a report or memorandum that lays out the background and advantages and disadvantages of various courses of action which address the issue that has been raised is to define and circumscribe the subject of inquiry. Advisers must ask themselves and their principal how deep and how broad the investigation needs to be, whether the problem as formulated by the principal is the "correct" problem or, for example, is part of a broader question that needs to be addressed, whether to be "politically" realistic—that question does not apply solely to actions involving government—or whether to be "visionary" and, as critics might term it, "unrealistic." This is not a matter of "letting the chips fall where they may." Advisers do not seek to recommend action without considering the impact of their actions. Rather, it is a matter of the constraints one believes have been placed or self-imposed on one's advice. It is tempting, but incorrect, to believe that adequate guidance can and will be provided by the decision maker who asks the initial question. That may occur, but my experience suggests that would be somewhat unusual. After all, more often than not, the principal knows less about the subject of inquiry than his or her advisers. He or she may hold strong opinions, biases, and presuppositions, all of which have to be taken into account, but may have devoted far less serious thought to the issue than has the staff. Thus, the definition of the problem is no trivial matter. It cannot be dealt with as is so often done in question and answer sessions after a lecture. Then the speaker may say, "That's a very good question" and proceed to avoid a response while talking around the subject. The adviser needs to do far better than that.

I encountered this issue in a serious way during the summer and early fall of 1964, a few short months before the November election that pitted President Lyndon Baines Johnson against Senator Barry Goldwater. Sometime in July I received a phone call from Kermit Gordon, then the director of the Bureau of the Budget. I had known Kermit from the time that I joined the staff of the Council of Economic Advisers during the summer of 1961 when Walter Heller (chairman), James Tobin, and Kermit were the three Council members. Then, as now, the Council was a small organization and staff and Council members intersected on a continuing basis and worked closely together. That was especially true of the drafts of the President's Economic Message and Council's Economic Report which, at that time, were released around mid-January. We lived through the preparation of these documents which were the administration's major report concerning the economy's performance in the year that had just concluded and its statement concerning the economic outlook and priorities for the coming year. For those who might be involved in similar exercises in which something they have drafted needs to be circulated for comment to many others in different agencies and departments and who want to minimize the number of comments they have to deal with, a word of advice may be useful. Provide a time that appears adequate for a careful reading—you owe that to your colleagues—but pick a time that makes it difficult to respond in an extremely detailed manner within the relevant time period. We sent out the first draft just before Christmas asking for a rapid turn around and the next draft, the revision, just before New Year's again requesting a rapid response. Our timing proved effective in reducing comments on minor matters.

In a sense this was analogous to what we knew as the Ted Sorenson rule, so named after its author who was special counsel and adviser to President Kennedy. That rule, a useful one for any decision maker or policy adviser who sends memoranda to others for comment, can be stated quite simply: "Don't write marginal comments such as 'This doesn't scan well,' or 'There must be a better way to make this point,' or similar editorial remarks. If you don't like a word or a phrase or the way the argument was put, rewrite it. I want you to provide substitute language, not 'sidebar' comments or queries." I once spotted a word I believed inappropriate and unacceptable in a presidential message and, knowing it wasn't enough to point that out, spent half a day searching for a word that had the same alliteration but was more acceptable. Of course, that rule reduced the number of trivial or unintelligible comments.

The staff and Council members were a family: when one leaves the office together with others at 3:00 AM it does make for a close relationship. We debated every economic idea and argued—sometimes it seemed interminably—over the nuances of every word: should we write "wage-price guidelines" which might imply a certain rigidity in the desired relationship between wages and prices and, therefore, suggested some type of government intervention if prices rose more rapidly than wages or would we be better served by a somewhat "looser" formulation that implied flexibility, as in "wage-price guideposts?" How might we best resist those who wanted us to set a very low unemployment target, one which we felt would exacerbate inflationary pressures and was "unrealistic?" Could we finesse the issue by stating a target rate higher than that preferred by our colleagues in the Labor Department and calling it "an interim" target, something that we could aim for and that we would have to "pass through" on our way to anything lower? One of the benefits of the process was that the various members of the staff came to more than just know each other.

I left the Council in 1963 having completed the two-year stint that was the normal tour of duty for those on leave from a university position. As it turned out, I did not return to Chapel Hill and instead moved to the Brookings Institution, which at the time was considered a centrist/liberal think tank. I claimed that I did not have "Potomac Fever," but it was clear that staying in Washington would permit me to continue my involvement with and relationship—even if on an informal basis—with government. Thus, I was "in the neighborhood" when Kermit called to ask that I join a small group of individuals who were being asked to serve on the president's health task force and who would prepare a health care agenda that LBJ would want to consider if, as expected, he would win the November election. Neither the membership of the group or even its formation would be made public. Thus we would be spared any lobbying by various individuals and organizations with a desire to influence our deliberations. The president wanted to win the election, examine our agenda and those of the other task forces that were being appointed, set his priorities and then face the various political pressures in favor of this or that piece of legislation.

I agreed to serve on the task force and to participate actively in its work. I did not inquire who else was asked to join in the effort or even who would chair the group. As it turned out most of the eight members were individuals with whom I had worked or who were known to me. I was not surprised to find that the chairperson as well as almost all of the participants was a physician/administrator.

Shortly after the group was constituted and had held its first meeting we were told we would have an opportunity to meet with the president who would provide us with useful guidance and context for our activity. Needless to say, we all looked forward to

that meeting. It was probably the case that every one of the committee members had met a president—though, perhaps, only at a
reception in a receiving line after a White House conference—but
even so it hardly was an everyday occurrence. In addition to the
substantive discussion that we looked forward to and that we believed would be helpful in our deliberations, meeting the president
and perhaps especially this activist president who was leading the
War on Poverty and helping build the Great Society was an exciting
prospect. And so it was that on a given day we found ourselves in
a small room in the White House waiting to be called in to meet
the president of the United States.

Much to our surprise instead of being called into his office,
Lyndon Baines Johnson entered—nay, strode—into the anteroom. I
rather suspect that even in the midst of the confusion, my colleagues
were as taken aback as I by what a large man he was. Of course,
we had seen countless photographs of him and had watched him on
television. We knew he was big. Yet, it was when he towered over
us or when he had our hand in his grasp as he quite unnecessarily
introduced himself, that we fully realized how large and impos-
ing—even intimidating—he was. He moved through the room and
each of us introduced himself. As I write "himself," I am reminded
and struck by how much America has changed over the last decades.
There was no woman on the task force (or for that matter among
the aides and assistants to the task force members), a situation that
is best ascribed not to the fact that there were no qualified women,
but to the fact that those who came up with the list of members
simply didn't think of, and did not think it necessary to think of,
potential women members. It is also worth noting that though we
were meeting in the midst of the Civil Rights revolution, the task
force had no minority members. We were a small group of white
males who provided evidence that the "old boy's" network was
very much alive.

In many, but not all respects that network is still alive, but fortunately is not as "hale and hearty." While some who choose committee members, speakers for symposia or managerial employees
automatically consider women and minorities for selection, there
remain others who do not. But in today's world no one can easily

overlook the issue. Considering "others" may not come naturally, but it comes and when it does so it enriches the policy discussions. It is not that some "quota" has been reached or that a public relations debacle has been avoided, but that new inputs from people with different experiences have been added. Those who would ignore including "others" will be reminded to evaluate non-traditional candidates and may be required to submit the names of women and others who have been rejected and the reasons why. Over time—and it does take time—thinking of "others" will become a habit, a pattern of behavior. I have little doubt that had Kermit told his assistant to submit the names of women and minority candidates who had been considered and rejected, individuals from those groups would have joined the committee. He didn't think of it and I regret to say that even if I noticed at the time, I didn't speak up. As I look back on our discussions, I conclude that the committee undoubtedly lost useful inputs from members who would have been sensitive to issues and matters we overlooked.

In striding through the small room the president filled the space and, in fact, forced some of us to try to get out of his way so that he could move through the room and meet others. Indeed, I found that since I had been closest to the door through which LBJ entered and the first one who had been greeted and who had introduced himself, I worked especially hard to get to other side of the room and "out of the way." But as the president continued his advance he soon was once again standing in front of me. As he towered over me, he enveloped my hand in his, introduced himself, and waited for me to do the same, I realized that, not surprisingly, our encounter only two or three minutes earlier was a much bigger event for me than it had been for him. Appropriately, I'd go home and tell my children I'd met the president; appropriately he wouldn't tell Lucy and Linda that he'd met that fellow from Brookings, Rashi Fein.

Far more important than the excitement of the meeting, was the president's message. He was very explicit that he did not want us to give him an agenda constrained by what we believed to be politically feasible. He reminded us that we weren't politicians, but that he was. Our job was to tell him what the nation needed so that we might all be proud of America's health performance *over the coming decades*. His job was to see that the proper legislation would be enacted so that the nation might reach the goals we put before him. He made it abundantly clear that he wanted us to tell him what legislation was required in order to create a better and fairer America, one that met its citizens' needs and fulfilled his and our aspirations. He stressed that he had the responsibility to assure that such legislation would be enacted. We were to dream; he was to translate those dreams into reality.

It is important to remember that the reference to a long-term strategy—where our nation should be twenty or thirty years hence—was articulated during the summer of 1964. At the time Medicare which had been discussed and debated for years as an important but limited program that would insure hospital care but that did not cover physicians' services had not yet been enacted. Medicaid, the program that pays for health care for some, though not all, of the poor was not even on the public agenda. Nor were various other health related programs with which America was to become familiar. Thus, the opportunity—indeed, the requirement—that we "think big," that we dream and leave the political judgments to LBJ, was both exciting and challenging. After all, we were working for a president who was a master of the political process. His legislative record both as majority leader of the Senate and in the months following the assassination of President Kennedy provided ample evidence that things could happen. We believed that we would not be preparing a document "for the files," but one for *action*.

Nevertheless, later, when we gathered to discuss our response to the charge that the president had put before us, it became clear that not everyone was prepared to seize the opportunity to think in long range and non-political terms or to "think big." This was made explicit by our chairman who took note of what the president had requested and then stated that nevertheless we had to be "practical" and "realistic." He argued that it would be silly to suggest so many legislative initiatives or such big changes that we would become a laughing stock. In spite of the president's cautionary note that we were not necessarily able politicians, we were to behave as if we had the requisite credentials. Our recommendations had to be "responsible." Most task force members agreed, though two of us protested that we would be misleading the president if we tempered our recommendations by the criterion of so called "realism," especially since we had little idea of what was and what was not realistic. We felt that if the group began its deliberations in an atmosphere of caution and "respectability" we would be unresponsive to the presidential charge. We feared the president would believe we were sketching a picture of a better America, what we believed America should and could be in a few decades when, in fact, we were adopting a very short-term perspective. I suggested—though not very seriously—that if we chose that path we needed to tell the president that we were not responding to his request, but had revised it to meet what we thought he should have asked. My colleagues gave that approach a cool reception.

In retrospect, it seems clear that I neglected to consider the forces that played upon the various people around the table. There is an important lesson in that observation for every policy adviser who is part of a group: think about and evaluate the next person's agendas and the multiple agendas around the table. I behaved as if all that I had to do to make my case and win the day was to present a convincing argument that we should be responsive to the presidential request. I ignored the fact that a number of members were not free agents. At least one influential member had very close ties to a high executive branch official who believed that the long run is made up of intermediate runs and the intermediate run consists of short run actions and, thus, that the latter should be our focus. Years later, this member apologetically told me that he reported all our deliberations and cleared the positions he advanced with his friend. Others were, or represented, administration officials with important administrative responsibilities in the health field, responsibilities that added immeasurably to their knowledge base, but that may have led them to place a premium on "feasibility." Nor did I take account of conflicts of interest: would members advocate new programs, however meritorious, that impinged on programs they were directing or on tasks for which they were responsible? I ignored a cardinal rule: know as much as possible about your colleagues, the other committee members. That knowledge may help structure a compelling argument.

The task force did produce a report. We recommended a laundry list of initiatives. Like most laundry lists, it had a certain pedestrian quality. Most recommendations called for increased appropriations for and expansion of already existing programs or the establishment of "study commissions." Worthwhile and beneficial as increased appropriations or new deliberative bodies might have been, they would not have brought much change to existing patterns of financing, organization, or distribution of health services. They could hardly have served as the framework of a "Health Message" from the president to the congress. The clerk who would have read the message—indeed, even the president if he delivered it—would not have inspired his audience. Our document could hardly be translated into a call to action nor was it a compelling description of a coherent program that would alter the trajectory of American health care. Indeed, the only novel and somewhat daring recommendation called for increased funding for construction of ambulatory health care facilities for "comprehensive group practice," a proposal designed to deal with the long-standing discrimination against physicians who practiced in a prepaid group practice setting.

Certainly, when we came to the discussion of the financing of care our rhetoric about health care needs and about the large number of persons who could not pay for medical care services was not matched by the vision that the president had called for. We supported a social insurance program for hospital care and home health care services for the aged (essentially what had already been proposed as Medicare and what, when it was enacted as part of a broader and more comprehensive program, came to be Medicare Part A), a program of limited assistance that would help states finance nursing home care for poor aged individuals who encompassed a part—but only a part—of today's Medicaid program, a program of limited assistance for poor children, and the appointment of a "committee of experts" to examine such matters as the impact of the medical expense deduction in the Internal Revenue code, the feasibility of protection against catastrophic medical expenses, and other measures that might assist low-income families in meeting medical care expenses.

We should have been embarrassed that, having been asked to be visionary, the task force recommended the establishment of additional task forces. After all, as policy advisers we were not providing especially helpful advice when, without providing any options that needed fleshing out, we suggested that what the president needed to do was to call on other policy advisers. Two of us asked for and, though it was considered unusual and "bad form," were finally given the opportunity to add addenda and recommendations that went beyond those in the consensus document. In each case, the statement recommended the enactment of a fully comprehensive national health insurance program providing for universal coverage and based on social insurance principles.

The fact is that LBJ was correct in telling us we were not good politicians or assessors of what was feasible. That is evident when one considers that the various initiatives we recommended and more, many more, were enacted within the year. For example, we had limited our recommendation for the aged—the Medicare population—only to hospital benefits and, on grounds of "realism" not reflecting real needs, had not dared recommend coverage for physician services. Yet, when Medicare was enacted it included a Part B that dealt with those very services. Nor, even though we had been enjoined to think in terms of a two to three decade time horizon, did we recommend that disabled persons be covered by the Medicare program. Yet, such coverage was added to the original Medicare program within a very few years. Similarly, we had recommended the establishment of a committee to study the problems of the low income population and had not considered or urged a program similar to the one that came to be known as Medicaid. Though we were supposed to look twenty years into the future, as a committee we had nothing to say about universal health insurance, a subject which though it failed to be enacted did receive serious consideration within the decade.

Nevertheless, it should be noted that apparently our limited vision had no untoward consequences. Our report did not exert a restraining influence on this activist president. Under LBJ'S guidance—and with inputs from a dedicated and knowledgeable staff of civil servants who collectively had greater detailed information and knowledge than our committee—Congress enacted a "bumper crop" of health legislation. In addition to physician and hospital benefits under Medicare and Medicaid, Congress authorized and appropriated sums to provide assistance to community mental health centers, Office of Economic Opportunity Neighborhood Health Centers, Head Start and children and youth projects, (including their health components), comprehensive health planning, regional medical programs (with emphasis on heart, cancer, and stroke), multi-county demonstration health facilities, public health formula grants, grants for health services demonstration projects, training grants for the expansion of the supply of nurses and other allied health professionals, as well as support for medical, dental, optometry, pharmacy, and veterinary education. The fact that our recommendations were modest did not preclude the successful adoption of a much richer legislative agenda. In that sense "we did no harm." Regrettably, we also did little "good." Our limited—and, as it turned out, incorrect—view of realism triumphed over vision.

I digress to reassure the reader who is somewhat confused by that list of new programs, the reader who says, "I follow politics; I keep up with current events. How could there have been so much legislation in so short a period? That doesn't happen; that's not the way the system works." That is a reasonable reaction for someone too young to have participated in or witnessed political events some forty years ago and it is especially the case when one recognizes that in addition to health legislation there were similar broad initiatives in other fields such as education, labor, income maintenance and, of course, in the area of civil rights. To offer complete explanations for this phenomenon would take us far afield. It must suffice to note that it really did occur and that it took place under the leadership of a president who, though tragically remembered for the war in Vietnam, fought a war on poverty and tried to build a "great society." Nor can we overlook the contributions made by civil servants, a term that has been sneered at and replaced by the negative word "bureaucrat" in recent years. The civil service provides the institutional memory and the knowledge base that every president and all political appointees must rely upon. Policy makers or advisers who ignore those government employees will inevitably accomplish much less than would otherwise be the case. Regrettably, as presidents have run their campaigns against "Washington" and have denigrated its public servants, the negative impact on the civil service has been considerable and we shall have to rebuild if it is to achieve its former levels of competence.

The awareness that much can be accomplished even in the absence of a crisis such as the Great Depression is important. It may help buttress a hope, perhaps even a belief that we once again can recapture a spirit of optimism about our ability to enact and implement legislation designed to advance well-being. In turn that belief can lead to action.

It is clear that I felt and still feel that we had not served the President as well as we might have because, in not delivering what he had asked for, we may have confused him and his staff. It is not that we did not offer a detailed agenda for action; we did not even sketch the "big picture." Our definition of "realism" was far too limited. We had been asked to be "radical" and, as so often turns out to be the case on committees, had chosen to be "respectable." I believe that a very similar phenomenon can be found in today's discussions of health insurance. One often hears colleagues state privately—and on rare occasions even publicly—that a tax-based program that provided all of us with nationally defined comprehensive health insurance benefits with only a minimal administrative role for insurance companies, say, something like a "Medicare for All" approach, would be a more efficient and effective way to reach universal coverage than other alternatives. They recognize that today's employment based health insurance system negatively impacts price-competition among firms whose employees have different demographic characteristics and medical care needs. Nor does employment based insurance provide for the needs of those who work for low wage and low profit employers or for those who are not working and are not covered by Medicare or Medicaid.

Yet, even as they decry existing arrangements and have little hope that the employment linked "broken" approach can be salvaged and built upon, many of those colleagues take today's politics as given and dismiss the "Medicare for All" or "single-payer" approach on the grounds that it is too radical, lacks sufficient political support, and simply isn't politically possible. They conclude that if they want to be part of the debate about reform of the health care system they must temper their views, The consequence, of course, is that we do not benefit from a presentation of the full range of options because the choices that are offered are circumscribed by political judgments which may be faulty. I believe that those who dismiss the single-payer approach, not on analytic grounds but because it is "unrealistic" might well have dismissed the existing Medicare program on a similar basis. They would have been wrong, but would have felt at home on our task force.

Nevertheless, policy advising isn't as simple as all that. It is possible to read one's self out of the debate and to have one's ideas dismissed as foolish, not in keeping with the real world, too far out. The adviser who doesn't entertain any idea unless it is "realistic" and clearly "doable" may accomplish less than is possible. It is also true, however, that the adviser who advocates positions that are consistently out of keeping with her or his principal's views may soon need to find other employment. There is another side to the issue of "advice untrammeled by political judgment." Once again, as in so many aspects of policy advice, there is the need for balance. That was driven home by an incident that took place when I was serving on the staff of the Council of Economic Advisers.

With only a very few exceptions staff members of the CEA were accountable for keeping up with developments and providing analyses of events dealing with their particular area of responsibility: industrial organization, international trade, labor issues, and so forth. Policy issues were most often discussed in meetings involving one or two Council members and only those staff members who were expert on the issues at hand. Most of the general staff meetings related to administrative matters, decisions about the Annual Report, and other issues that cut across all areas. On rare occasions a meeting was arranged to solicit the views of the staff and perhaps of a few other economists who also "worked for the President" on an issue on which no one of us had sufficient expertise. One such meeting took place when we had been asked what we would recommend as the appropriate administration posture on the matter of patent and royalty policy under the Kefauver drug bill. Senator Estes Kefauver of Tennessee had long been interested in the economic behavior of drug companies and in federal economic and regulatory policy on pharmaceuticals. Part of the legislation that Kefauver proposed was designed to increase price competition in the drug field by changes in patent protection. Our views on the amendments had been solicited by Wilbur Cohen, assistant secretary for legislation in the Department of Health, Education, and Welfare (HEW). That, in itself, was unusual. Wilbur had long and extensive experience in government and years of involvement with the issues that HEW faced. That and the fact that he was assisted by a knowledgeable and highly motivated staff meant that he seldom felt the need to turn to the CEA for comment on issues either of substance or politics.

The issue of patent protection and royalties under the Kefauver drug legislation, however, was unlike any of the other policy questions Wilbur had tackled. Perhaps he felt that this purely economic issue belonged to the CEA which surely would have the expertise to analyze the implications of Kefauver's initiative. Perhaps he also wanted to avoid taking sides on an issue that involved Kefauver and the president since they had an unusual relationship. In 1956 the Democratic nominee for president, Adlai Stevenson, threw the choice of a vice presidential nominee to the delegates at the party convention. Kefauver defeated Kennedy and secured the nomination. In any event, because of the nature of the request, the absence of sufficient expert staff, and Walter's desire to feel more comfortable with whatever advice the CEA would offer, the chairman took the relatively unusual step of convening a staff meeting.

As Walter went around the room soliciting comments and offering each staff member and guest an opportunity to present his or her views, it became clear that we all were of a similar mind. Though some participants felt more strongly than others, there was unanimous agreement with the proposition that the administration should support that part of the Kefauver proposal requiring that drug manufacturers who held a patent allow competing firms to produce the patented drug and pay the patent holder a royalty. The cost of producing a drug was so low that even with the royalty payment the new entrant could undercut the price charged by the firm that had a monopoly. Competition would benefit consumers by helping to reduce the escalation in the cost of pharmaceuticals.

After soliciting the views of staff the chairman turned to the Council members who till then had remained silent. When he called on Kermit Gordon who outside of Walter himself was the one remaining person who had not spoken, Kermit surprised us all by presenting a different point of view. He began with a story that some of us knew but had either forgotten or whose applicability to the matter before us had escaped our notice. He recounted that when the Second World War ended, President Truman announced that meat rationing would need to continue for a limited time. After all, the fact that the war was over did not increase the supply of meat available and the president felt that the nation should continue to make meat available in what had come to be viewed as a "fair" manner. Collective sacrifice was necessary till the nation had completed its shift to a peacetime footing. Furthermore, absent any short-run supply response, removal of rationing would lead to rapid and large price increases that would feed inflationary pressures.

As Kermit told it, the ranchers were angered by the president's decision since, given the limited supply of meat, the removal of rationing would have enabled them to reap a "windfall" as a result of the significant increases in price. They decided to withhold cattle from market and to blame the administration for creating an even greater meat "shortage." The strategy worked: less meat came to market and the public's frustration and resentment were visited upon the president rather than the ranchers. Presumably, it was he who had caused the shortage by maintaining rationing and not giving the market free reign.

The argument that Kermit presented built upon that experience. He agreed that if the Kefauver drug bill were adopted, firms that had to pay royalties to produce the patented product would be able to undercut the prices charged by those who had developed the drugs. That would be beneficial. The difficulty was that, in turn, even if the royalty payment were large, the old-line "research" companies who had underwritten the major research efforts that had resulted in the patentable new drug would claim that, unable to "receive the rewards for innovation"—surely, a well-chosen more felicitous phrase than "to reap monopoly profits"—they could no longer afford to sponsor pharmaceutical research. The federal government would be unable to make up for the shortfall in research on new drugs by sufficiently increasing the efforts of the National Institutes of Health. The American public would have to choose whom to blame: government for taking actions that inhibited research (never mind the large expenditures by pharmaceutical companies on efforts to promote drug utilization) or the drug companies for constraining competition and maximizing monopoly profits. Kermit argued that, given American attitudes toward government and toward the "free" market, the public would blame government in general and the administration in particular. Thus, support for Kefauver was fraught with political danger.

The story was compelling. It turned the tide. The enthusiasm for the Kefauver drug bill evaporated. Our earlier economic analysis had been trumped by political analysis.

I do not know how our advice to the president was couched. Perhaps we presented the economics and added a warning about the possible political dynamics; perhaps we dropped the economics and focused entirely on the political mine-fields. I do remember that I was very disturbed that the Council of Economic Advisers might be offering political advice which was not labeled as such, advice that the recipient would assume was based on economics. I came to the office early the next morning, early enough to intercept Kermit before he began his day's work and his round of meetings. I suggested that we may have done the White House a disservice by tainting our economic analysis with politics. Perhaps there was someone in the president's inner circle who had thought that "sticking it to the drug companies" was good politics. Perhaps there were political considerations we did not know about. Perhaps it was important to the president's power and influence in the Senate to support Kefauver. Perhaps decision makers now felt they had to follow what they assumed was the CEA's advice based on economic analysis.

Kermit listened carefully and proceeded to put my concerns into a wider context. He told me that he had a friend who recently had assumed a high position in the Department of State. He was an important economic adviser to the secretary and had taken the position only after he was assured that he could "call the shots as he saw them" and offer advice not sullied by the grubby world of politics. Indeed, that characterized his memoranda; his was the voice of pure economics. Now, a few months later, he found that no one was reading his memoranda. The memos were out of touch with the real world of Washington and were not necessarily consonant with the goals and aims of the administration. The point, Kermit stated, was that one should not divorce economic analysis and recommendations from their context, that economic policy was rooted in time, place, institutional considerations, and values. The effective adviser was the one who balanced the various considerations, a point I should have recognized. After all, I had received my doctorate majoring in political economy not in economics. Furthermore, I was well aware that while council members respected Milton Friedman as an economist, we did not consult with him. Instead we regularly consulted with Paul Samuelson with whom—among others—we shared common goals. We sought advice from many parties and welcomed differences of opinion. But those differences related to mechanisms, methods, policies to achieve specified goals and the impacts of such policies, not the aims, objectives, and the goals of the administration.

In a telling comment Ted Sorenson has written: "When Walter Heller told me that his team of economic advisors' recommendation on a particular issue had been altered to take political considerations into account, I scolded him, telling him that the president and I could make the political calculations, and wanted from him and his colleagues their best and most objective substantive recommendations." But, before we conclude that I was correct and Kermit wrong, Sorenson adds, "Yet, in the larger sense of the term "politics," all of us on the president's staff knew that we were in part the president's political advisors and that the White House is inherently a political institution.[2]

What then are policy advisers left with as they consider both the need for political realism and the need for vision? It would be well if there were a formula one could follow that assured the correct weight for each of the many variables an adviser should consider. There isn't. Advising is an art not a science. What can be taught is that a narrow focus in which the economist is no more than an economist and in which every adviser limits his or her concerns and analyses only to their narrow "home" discipline is not likely to serve the interests of those receiving that advice. At the same time what must also be taught is that there are disciplinary bases and the economist and representative of other disciplines should not encompass so broad a focus that all advice is blurred.

The effective adviser somehow combines "realism" and "vision," knowledge of her or his discipline with a rich knowledge of other field of inquiry. The effective adviser is both a theorist and an institutionalist. Perhaps the effective adviser needs to embody some of the skills of a master politician. Of course, that kind of versatility most often needs to be gained through experience rather than through formal education—which increasingly is described—unfortunately, accurately—as "training." As the various disciplines are becoming ever more specialized, we find that our educational institutions are "training" economists, sociologists, and political scientists rather than educating social scientists. That this does not meet the full needs of policy analysis has been recognized by others as, for example, the Robert Wood Johnson Foundation which provides post-doctoral fellowships designed to enlarge the skills and cross-discipline-cutting knowledge base of scholars who are interested in moving into the health policy field.

A final and important word is in order. In his volume on President Kennedy, Ted Sorenson writes that, on occasion, JFK preferred a compromise to no bill at all and offers some examples to support that observation. One example he cites relates to the Kefauver drug bill. He reports that the president was convinced that including changes to patent protection would have blocked the entire bill and recognized that a substitute bill was necessary since Kefauver could not publicly abandon his long standing support for patent revisions. With Kefauver's knowledge, the president prevailed upon Senator

Eastland to submit a drug reform bill that did not contain the patent proposals, but was even stronger on other aspects related to consumer protection.[3] I doubt that any of us at the staff meeting were privy to these political and personal considerations. Perhaps that is yet another argument for the professional economist to exhibit appropriate humility about her or his credentials as a politician and give more weight to the potential contribution that she or he might make in practicing one's discipline. One thing is clear: the person seeking advice and the person offering it should understand the nature of the advice and the information and judgment on which it is based. The adviser who is asked to offer economic advice should not "smuggle in" his or her political assessment. If such assessment is appropriate, advisers should behave as if their advice is covered by a "Truth in Labeling" act that informs the principal what role the adviser is playing and what discipline or set of experiences informs the advice offered.

I do not imply, however, that the adviser's task is solely to respond to the specific question asked and to limit the answer to the narrow issue that he or she has been asked to address. An adviser who understands and has worked with a principal should feel comfortable in suggesting a reformulation of the request and in pointing out that dealing with that reformulated question might be more informative. It is akin to the relationship that I had with the owner of the local hardware store a few blocks from our home. Though the small local establishment charged a bit more, I frequented it, perhaps because at the larger chain store the help knew little more than where to find the various kinds of merchandise—the hammers are in aisle four and the screwdrivers in six. I learned that at the smaller family owned store the correct approach involved my describing the problem I had and what I was trying to accomplish and relying on the assessment of the owner to tell me what I needed. Quite often it wasn't "this" or "that," but something I didn't even know existed. So, too, with those who seek policy advice. They need to share the problem—not their attempt at a partial answer—with their advisers and failing that, their advisers need to behave as my hardware store owner did when he encouraged a reformulation of the question.

Asking the Correct Question

Sometimes the reformulation of the question, the suggestion that there is a broader issue that needs to be addressed, is of such consequence that it has a great impact and is long remembered. The reformulation entails a learning experience, a lesson that has meaning far beyond the limited issue raised in the substitution of the new question for the old. An example of what I mean occurred in a classroom at Harvard Medical School some forty years ago. I have not forgotten the student or the conversation.

I came to Harvard Medical School during the summer of 1968. At Harvard, "officialdom" often says that one is "called to Harvard," but as the graduate of another university, I found, and still find, the seriousness with which the institution took, and takes, itself a bit off-putting. So I had "come" after spending some nine years on the faculty of the University of North Carolina and the immediate previous seven years in Washington, D.C. The first two plus years of those seven were on the staff of the Council of Economic Advisers during the John F. Kennedy administration. The next five were as a member of the Economics Program at the Brookings Institution.

During the years I had spent both in and out of government I had been involved in dealing with and, on occasion, helping to develop public policy initiatives in the fields of education, health, welfare, and social security. These were the traditional agenda of the federal Department of Health, Education, and Welfare. I had also dealt with issues concerning civil rights, poverty and the distribution of income, the agenda of many agencies and departments, but especially of the Office of Economic Opportunity which was established during President Lyndon Johnson's administration as part of his War on Poverty and quest for the Great Society, and, as well, programs related to labor force issues and manpower retraining, matters of direct concern to the Department of Labor. I suppose that my public policy interests could be subsumed under the heading: the "do-good" programs. While at Brookings I wrote a book on the "doctor shortage"[4] and was involved in a number of other health-related activities.

My interests and experiences in the health arena were instrumental in bringing me to Harvard to join the faculties of the Harvard Medical School and the John F. Kennedy School of Government. I welcomed the opportunity to relocate. I wanted to return to teaching and I wanted to get out of Washington, a city that was consumed—in almost a pathological way—by the Vietnam War. I could recall earlier dinner parties where guests had avoided bringing up Vietnam lest the discussion grow so heated that the host and hostess would be embarrassed. Now it seemed that at the parties we attended the guests vied with each other to determine who abhorred Johnson the most. I knew there was no escape—nor should there have been—from discussions of the war. Still, I believed that if one left Washington, one could escape the pathology of hatred, that one could see Johnson as a tragic figure rather than as the embodiment of evil.

One of my many Washington experiences while at Brookings was participating in and reacting to the thrust of President Lyndon Baines Johnson's directive that all departments of government develop rigorous analytic efforts to assess and evaluate existing policies and to justify program initiatives. These efforts often involved approaches such as benefit-cost analysis, the technique that attempted to quantify all of the various benefits that a program might yield as well as the various costs that the program might incur. Benefits and costs could be compared because they were measured using a "common denominator," most often, dollars.

This approach, increasingly applied to issues in water resource management, fit well with the analytic thought patterns of economists—and economists became increasingly important on the Washington scene in the early 1960s. It was the very same approach that most, if not all of us had learned in our basic micro-economic courses. In considering how an individual might choose to spend his or her income, we had been taught that the individual presumably considered the satisfaction that might be derived from the last dollar of expenditure and adjusted expenditure choices so that they would maximize the total units of satisfaction. One would spend a dollar for French fries rather than for a coke or a newspaper if the satisfaction attained from the fries exceeded that provided by the alternatives. It seemed to make sense, though as students some of us observed that many individuals—including ourselves—didn't appear to weigh the various alternatives as carefully as was suggested, that occasionally we were impulse purchasers. We were told that, if true, that was because some of us preferred "impulse buying" having determined that the benefit of additional consideration did not measure up to the cost of that thought process. Thus by definition whatever the outcome one could argue that the consumer was always weighing alternatives, even the alternative of weighing alternatives. Tautologies are powerful.

Substitute the word "benefit" for "satisfaction" and one had a familiar guide to public policy choices: one should assess benefits and their relation to costs and appropriate dollars for various programs in a manner that maximized the benefits attained. Although not part of the process of formal decision-making, this approach had a long history.[5] Even as early as 1667 Sir William Petty had calculated how much it would cost to transport individuals out of London during a plague and compared that with the number of lives saved as a consequence. Using what he calculated as the "monetary value of a life," Petty concluded that moving people out of harm's way was a worthwhile "investment." There was a rich three-hundred-year history of intellectual effort to measure the economic value of human beings—most often as reflected by wages and incomes which presumably reflected their productivity—and the monetary benefits and costs of various human activities. This literature included studies in the health field, in education, in migration policy (host countries gained through migration, especially through migration of well-educated individuals who would be especially productive), and even whether war was a worthwhile "investment." Thus, it was "demonstrated" that though the Prussians won the Franco-Prussian war, when one translated the costs in human life and casualties into monetary terms, the Prussians had made a poor "investment."

Given my interests, as well that of the students, part of my course on "Economic Factors in the Organization and Financing of Health Care" was devoted to the presentation of the analytic thought pattern that could be used in an effort to maximize societal benefits associated with health programs financed by government or the not-for-profit sector, say, hospitals. The topic was not some mere exercise in esoteric thought about the allocation of resources. Students saw its considerable relevance to what they could observe in the medical care system they encountered. With the implementation of Medicare and Medicaid in 1966 and guaranteed payment on behalf of individuals who previously had little or no insurance coverage, hospitals, perhaps especially teaching hospitals, had embarked on major capital construction projects.

Yet, even as hospitals were expanding their size and technical capabilities, neighborhood and community health centers operating with funds from the Office of Economic Opportunity, the "Pentagon" of the nation's War on Poverty, faced funding cut-backs as the War in Vietnam took precedence. The then director of the Massachusetts General Hospital (MGH), John Knowles, observed that within the shadows of the world-renowned MGH one could find the highest infant mortality in the city of Boston. The disconnect between the existing patterns of health expenditures and of health needs was evident and called for analysis. That analysis needed a framework and while different disciplines would have provided different frameworks—political scientists, for example, surely would have focused on the role of politics in decision making—I had been educated as an economist and utilized and provided the students with an economic framework. How were alternatives considered and weighed, how were resources allocated, how should they be allocated?

So it was that on a given day in the spring of 1969 or 1970 I was presenting the approach that tried to equate benefits at the margin and, thus, to maximize benefits the total expenditures would yield. I was doing so with some passion, not because of the economist's appreciation of the "beauty" of the analytical framework, but because the mode of analysis was the way to understand how, by shifting expenditures, we could do much more for the human condition even within the constraints of available resources. Of course, we all knew that there were political and methodological problems: in the political world funds might be available for some purposes and not for others; donors might be willing to sponsor research tied to a particular disease and uninterested in supporting operating expenses of centers for primary care; various benefits could not be translated into dollar denominators, might be overlooked or ignored because they could not be measured; costs might be under or over stated. Nevertheless, the lecture presumed that it was important that students become acquainted with the economist's way of thinking about choices.

A hand shot up, and even before I could finish my sentence the question came: "If you don't have the money to do all the good things, why don't you take $5 billion from the Pentagon?" In those days, some forty years ago, $5 billion was real money: today national health expenditures are about $2 trillion; in 1970 they were a "mere" $75 billion. Adding five billion, almost seven percent, would make a big difference. It was true that in my presentation I had compared the benefit that the marginal expenditure, the last dollar, would yield across various health programs. I had not weighed the benefits of health expenditures against those associated with expenditures for education, transportation, the myriad of government programs including those of the Pentagon or, for that matter, against the satisfactions and benefits derived from private consumption that might be generated by spending fewer government dollars and cutting taxes. Yet, that was not the thrust of the question. That spring Harvard students, like many college students elsewhere, as well as an increasing proportion of the American population, were disillusioned by the Vietnam war and were quite prepared to argue that Pentagon dollars were doing more harm than good. Surely those dollars could be more used productively if expended on health care.

My response was clear. While I might agree about moving $5 billion from the Pentagon to the health budget, the analytic problem would remain: on which health program or programs should I spend the now available $5 billion. After all, whatever the resources I had, it would still be incumbent on me to spend them in the ways that maximized total benefits. "Ah," the student replied. "I understand, but if you had the $5 billion you wouldn't be so up-tight about it." Advantage student. My reply lobbed the ball back: "True, but we don't have the $5 billion, so let me continue presenting the analysis." I wanted to get back to the "lesson plan" and, perhaps, to more familiar economic terrain.

But it wasn't that simple. "Fair enough, but I do have one more question. Do you know why you don't have the $5 billion?" I fear I may have been exceedingly condescending. After all I had come from Washington. The federal budget and the budget process were things I had dealt with. In largest measure the dinner conversation at home was heavily political and I prided myself on having a degree in political economy, not just economics. What, therefore, could this first-year student at Harvard Medical School teach me about analyzing government expenditures? "No, I don't know why I don't have the $5 billion. Tell me."

The answer came crisply and has bounced around in my head these many years. It has served to raise difficult questions about the allocation of a scarce resource: one's own time. It has served as an introduction to issues that every one wrestles with, whether consciously or in a less deliberate fashion. "The reason you don't have the $5 billion is that you and all those guys like you spend all your time worrying about the way to spend the last dollar and have no time or energy left to go after the $5 billion." It was as if the ball whizzed by me: point, game, set, and match. My question had been a simple one: from whom should I take some pie so that I might have more? The question was reformulated: "how do we expand the pie?" By broadening my inquiry, my student—think of her as my adviser—had served me exceedingly well.

The answer—if one spends all his or her time worrying about how to spend the last dollar there will be no time left to work at obtaining more dollars—is not really about economics. I believe a far more important and general point is involved: the choice we all must make is the degree to which we accept constraints and operate within them and the degree to which we attempt to alter and push back those constraints. And there is more: we must choose between the degree to which we spend our time, energy, and effort on tasks that fall within our professional domain—say, economic analysis about allocating health care resources—and attempts to balance those efforts with those of broad citizenship—say, political activity that might radically alter available resources and budgets.

The reason I have remembered both the student—a very bright young woman who did not just talk about making the world a better place, but who has spent her life doing just that by both how and to whom she delivers medical care—and our exchange is that I believe she was telling me something extraordinarily important about the choices all of us must make. What she told me and what numerous other events have reinforced is that if our democracy is to survive it is not enough to be an economist, a salesperson, an electrician. One also has to find the time to be engaged in the civic society, to be a citizen. That is important if we are to strengthen the community of which we are a part. It is also important for the well-being of the individual for it is as Oliver Wendell Holmes, Jr. stated, "I think that, as life is action and passion, it is required of a man that he should share the passion and action of his time at peril of having been judged not to have lived."[6]

Of course, not everyone would agree with the reformulated question and its implication. I know some young professionals in the academic community who have found the story interesting, but have disagreed with the message that I believe it holds. Perhaps, more correctly, they have agreed with the sentiments, but not with the operational consequences. They remind me of the demands that college and university departments place upon them, of the need to do research and publish, of the quest for tenure. They remind me of family obligations and the rewards that family brings. They assure me that civic engagement will come in due time—after they have made their mark and achieved their promotions, after the "kids" have grown up and are on their own—though they may well underestimate how long that will take. Till then, political action and involvement has to be left to others, presumably individuals who have fewer demands placed on their time and/or those who are professionally engaged in "politics."

But, of course, the day when one has made her or his mark and relax may never come: there will always be one more grant to seek, one more article to write, one more lecture to deliver, one more honor yet to be achieved. The "kids" will grow up, but the rewards of family "engagement," albeit taking different forms, will remain and tempt further postponement of community involvement. Furthermore, the "temporary" non-involvement can easily become a habit, a pattern, a way of life. I am certain that my student would have found a response that suggested that one would go after the five billion dollars but not until some time in the future deeply troubling and appropriately so. She might have been reminded of the chorus in the Joe Hill labor song:

> You will eat, bye and bye,
> In that glorious land above the sky;
> Work and pray, live on hay, You'll get pie in the sky when you die

As in so many matters involving choice, the quest has to be for balance. We must put bread on the table by doing our job and doing it well, but we must save some time to work at changing the world. That, too, is our task. We must be concerned with making the wisest choices within the constraints of time, income, and the various responsibilities all of us face, but we must save some time to push back on those constraints and increase our available options. That, too, is our job as it is of the responsible policy adviser. These tasks cannot be turned over to "professional" volunteers. They can't be left for the next person.

In the National Portrait Gallery in Washington there hangs a portrait of the great chemist Linus Pauling who was awarded the Nobel Prize in Chemistry in 1954 and the Nobel Peace Prize in 1962. Next to the portrait there is displayed a quotation from Pauling: "I could have accomplished a lot more science from 1945 to 1965. I decided...I ought to get scientists working for peace.... Scientists have an obligation to help fellow citizens make the right decisions." My student and Linus Pauling would have understood each other. The benefits of the various activities each of us might engage in have to be balanced and equated at the margin. The NIH researcher and the bus driver, the grade school teacher and the coal miner—all of us—have to participate in acts of citizenship.

Some Changes Take Time

In suggesting a range of policy options, consideration must be given to the series of steps and span of time necessary to implement fully the newly adopted policy. New data systems, administrative procedures, and enforcement provisions do not spring into being. System change proceeds in stages and each stage take time. As previously noted, providing too long a time span invites delay in implementation while too short a time invites confusion and potential failure. Furthermore, policy changes often involve changes in behavior of many affected parties including individuals who disagree with the purposes of the new policy and who may choose to be uncooperative and to resist change or, if they have the choice, to opt out of coverage. The policy adviser must ask: "how will the policy work on the ground, how many individuals will avoid or evade the new program, what slippage will there be in coverage?" Such questions are always of importance. If overlooked, taken for granted, or assumed away, the called for policy may have less impact, at least in the short run than might have been anticipated. Various experiences in Chapel Hill, North Carolina in the years following the Supreme Court decision on school desegregation in Brown v Board of Education of Topeka, Kansas serve to illustrate the importance of time in assessing the "implementation" issue.

My wife, Ruth, and I moved to Chapel Hill in the summer of 1952, slightly less than two years before the court decision. We knew that some considered Chapel Hill the "southern part of heaven" and had been told that it was an "oasis in the south." Frank Porter Graham, former president of the University of North Carolina from 1930 to 1949 when he was appointed to a vacant U.S. Senate seat—subsequently he was defeated in a racist primary when he ran for a full term in 1950—was considered a liberal even by the presumably more exacting standards of the north. He had built an outstanding and renowned public university and that was before its successes in basketball had added to its luster. It was reported that legislators often said words to the effect that "I don't agree with all the things that Dr. Frank is doing down there, but if he says he needs this money, let's give it to him."

Both Ruth and I had some understanding of southern customs and attitudes; we had lived in Baltimore, "a northern city with a southern exposure," for some years. We had encountered racial segregation at plays and musicals presented at Ford's Theatre and were very much aware that Ford's was applying a standard that reflected attitudes held by many members of the white community. Furthermore, as students at Johns Hopkins University, we were aware that at that time the university, and its students and faculty were essentially lily white and that a black Professor at Morgan State, who had been invited by a white member of the Hopkins faculty to lunch at the Hopkins faculty club, was refused service. True, at the next annual meeting the incumbent members of the board who set the policy were voted out of office by the club membership which included graduate students as well as faculty, but the changes that were coming were coming very slowly and were not seen as inexorable. Baltimore was a segregated city and Hopkins was part of Baltimore.

Furthermore, in addition to the Baltimore experience, Ruth had grown up in Washington, D.C. Though the nation's capital, it also was a southern city. Even in the first half-year plus of 1952 when I worked in Washington for President Truman's Commission on the Health Needs of the Nation, my fellow workers and I encountered segregation. There were four or five of us who dealt with health manpower issues. One of us was an African-American. Almost every day one of us (but never our African-American colleague) would say something like "It's time to go to lunch." Invariably, four days out of five, our African-American co-worker would say that he had a previous appointment, an errand to run, a job to finish, or offer some other reason that explained why he could not join us. The rest of us would then go out and head over to the inexpensive Chinese restaurant a short block or two away. Once a week our colleague would say that he was free and would be glad to come with us. He and we were aware that called for a change in venue. Since we knew—or believed—that the Chinese restaurant would not admit blacks, we had to head to the cafeteria at the Veteran's Administration or the one at the Association of University Women, both of which were open to all of us.

As I think back upon this I am struck by the fact that it apparently took us a long time to figure out that our colleague was reporting he couldn't join us when, more likely, he simply did not want to constrain our choice of a place to eat. I am also very much aware that we did frequent a restaurant that most probably—like many, if not most, restaurants in downtown Washington—engaged in discriminatory behavior. I am certain we would not have eaten there if there had been a sign in the window that proclaimed a "Whites Only" policy. Nor would we have crossed a NAACP picket line had there been one. But the corrosive, subtle, and non-explicit racism—the kind that was simply the way things were and didn't hit us in the face—though not acceptable, was "accepted." If nothing else this serves as a reminder of how easy it is for a member of the majority to be overwhelmed by the dominant culture and, after a time, not even notice the way things are. The minority, of course, cannot and dare not forget.

In some sense, therefore, Ruth and I were prepared—more correctly, thought we were—for Chapel Hill. We certainly were steeped in descriptions, some true, some stereotypes, of the south. Nevertheless, our knowledge of the south was akin to that of, say, anthropologists encountering a somewhat exotic culture for the first time, one they had read about, but had not seen first hand. At most we probably assumed that the south would be like Baltimore or Washington, only more so. But, the south was different. Discrimination was not as subtle and there seemed to be no pressure to hide it; it stared you in the face and could not be overlooked. The Raleigh-Durham air terminal, then housed in a long Quonset hut, had four rest rooms. I learned that when I entered and saw one marked "Men" and one "Women." Heading for the appropriate one, I encountered a third marked "Gentlemen" and a fourth "Ladies." Even a northerner could figure out what the distinctions meant.

Things were different in the new airport terminal built during the 1950s. There a door marked "Men" was visible from the lobby. Behind that door two other doors divided the clientele by race. I presume the same was true for women. The face of discrimination was hidden from general and public view. In October, 1961 students and others who had become aware that the terminal had been built, at least in part, with federal funds threatened to picket the arrival of President Kennedy who was to deliver a major address at Kenan Stadium at UNC unless the signs were removed. They were.

When the University hospital opened its doors in 1952 there was no signage, for example, on elevators, rest-rooms, and drinking fountains that distinguished between "white" and "colored." Chapel Hill was an oasis. But the desert invaded: signage did appear shortly after a legislator was hospitalized and discovered that the "appropriate" signs were missing. Those signs and other segregated facilities in hospitals disappeared throughout the South as an important and beneficial side-effect of the implementation of Medicare and the enforcement of federal civil rights statutes that prohibited the payment of federal dollars to segregated institutions.

Chapel Hill was an oasis, but an oasis in the South was still of the South. Nevertheless, when the school desegregation decision was promulgated in 1954, the community at large seemed to accept the fact that from then on things would be different, at least in the schools. The gas station on our corner did not take down the "White Only" sign, the movie theatre remained segregated, and the dairy bar would not seat African-Americans. Had some of the university administrators who, in 1952 when I came to Chapel Hill, used the term "nigra"—a variant that purposefully was sometimes difficult to distinguish from the N word—still been upon the scene they might well have continued to speak as they had spoken. Nevertheless, the university did desegregate. It did so slowly and "carefully," that is, by admitting an even number of African-Americans, thus making certain that white students did not have to share a dorm room with minority students, but desegregate it did. And the faculty, including those faculty members who did not refer to the "Civil War" or to the "War Between the States," but to the "War for Southern Independence" did try to adjust. In large measure they succeeded.

And that brings me to the encounter with a colleague on our faculty. An individual who was born and bred in the South, he was a professor of one of the disciplines in the school of business. He may, or may not have spent some time in the north or in the west, but, if so, very little had rubbed off. Intelligent and literate, he knew that the world was changing and may even have felt that the changes were appropriate as well as necessary. Yet, I am quite certain, that if he did so, that encompassed an intellectual rather than an emotional perspective. Even if in his mind he accepted desegregation, in his heart and surely in his visceral reactions he remained a son of the

South. One day, in conversation, he responded to something I said about southern attitudes toward race with a "But, Rashi, I'm trying. Believe me, I'm trying and I'm getting there and maybe some day I'll be there." I asked "What does that mean? What is it that you're trying? What does it mean you're getting there but, apparently, aren't there yet?" His answer, his very honest answer, was precise: "Look, I go swimming in the University pool almost every day. If I am in the water and a black student comes out of the locker room and heads toward the pool, I am very aware of my reaction, but I fight those reactions and stay in the pool. I don't get out. That's what I mean by progress, by 'I'm getting there.' Believe me, to stay in the water is no small thing; you don't understand that for me it's a very big change. But you ask what I mean when I say I'm not there yet, but I'm trying. That means that if I come out of the locker room to go into the pool and see that there's a black student already in the water, I stop and try and turn on my heel and go back to the locker room. I know it isn't logical, but it just isn't the same and so I'll swim later or some other day. But, believe me, I'm trying."

I have remembered what my colleague said and believe that he seemed to embody a combination of pride in how far he had come and anguish that he had not yet been able to go farther—though, perhaps, I exaggerate both the pride and anguish. I suppose that I remember it in part because of what I believed to be its honesty and specificity as well as his willingness to share a certain intimacy—we were colleagues not friends. I've also remembered it because it speaks to two issues: to the possibility for change in attitude that follows on change in behavior and environment and as well the need to recognize that change can come, but may require a kind of gestation time. It did take a decision by the Supreme Court of the United States—one should stop for a moment and not just read the two words "Supreme Court" that are so familiar that we overlook their significance, but read the single word "Supreme" and stop and consider its meaning: the *Supreme* court—to alter the environment and require changes in behavior. President Eisenhower stated that "you can't legislate morality." But we have learned that we can legislate behavior; it was Martin Luther King who stated that you "can legislate moral behavior."

Importantly, while we have known that changes in attitude will lead to changes in behavior, it is also the case that over time changes in behavior, even if under the force of law, may lead to changes in attitude. Nevertheless, while compulsory changes in environment and in behavior, as in admitting blacks to the university, can come relatively quickly, changing both attitudes and voluntary behavior—getting into and out of the swimming pool—takes longer.

Sometimes those who must deal with the implementation of public policy seem to believe that the variable called "time" need not be carefully considered, except, perhaps, in terms of the need to develop new administrative structures, hire new personnel, purchase computers, and so on and so forth. Decision makers and their advisers often fail to take account of the time required for "acceptance." Conversely, at other times, fearful of massive change, they allow an excess of time for new approaches to be implemented, inviting resistance and almost causing things to move so slowly that one can hardly discern changes in behavior and in attitudes. It may be that policies and legislation that are phased in with a predetermined time table may be more acceptable than things that are designed to happen either in "one fell swoop" or, as in "with all deliberate speed," at some unspecified future time. Does one adopt a "swim or sink" strategy or a "crawl before you walk" approach?

David Lloyd George stated that "The most dangerous thing in the world is to try to leap over a chasm in two jumps."[7] The visual image is striking and certainly compels a call for bold action. How, after all, can one rehabilitate the dysfunctional American health care system in tiny incremental steps? Is it not the case that the small actions, even if numerous, are swallowed up and negated by the system and culture in which they become imbedded, and, thus, may fail to add up to one big action. Nevertheless, visual images notwithstanding, "tiny," as in incremental, steps are not synonymous with "small" and certainly not with "fair sized." Nor is "a step now and we'll return to the issue again at a time unspecified," as is often implied in incremental steps, the same as a series of steps each of which is specified in advance and phased in at a predetermined time or at a predetermined trigger point.

While the issue of "what rate of speed," the "what and when" of policy may sound abstract, it has been a source of considerable tension in numerous public policy debates, including, and perhaps especially, the issue of universal health care. On one side have been those who have argued that the nation should adopt a program that moves from where we are to universal coverage in one leap. On the other hand were those who said that approach could and would not be accommodated by the American political system and in any case presumed an administrative capacity that was lacking. The first group was comprised of some academics and a few legislators. The second group—represented, for example, by President Carter and his allies in 1978-79—argued for taking a first step and revisiting the issue at some unspecified future time. In between was yet a third group led by Senator Kennedy that proposed the adoption of a phased approach, a step at a time but on a predetermined schedule. Even if both the administration's and the senator's positions had called for the same first step (and that was not the case), there was a vast political difference between the president's position that required a renewal of legislative debate whenever each subsequent step was considered and the senator's position that specified the what and when of future steps and that would have required a legislative debate to depart from that schedule.

There is no formula to which one can refer to ascertain the appropriate schedule for implementation of policies that call for large changes. But we should be aware that under the right conditions and with the right leadership even large changes can be implemented quickly. Medicare was debated for many years, finally enacted and signed into law on July 30, 1965 and fully implemented on July 1, 1966. In only eleven months we moved from a situation in there was no program covering services for seniors over sixty-five to a system that had enrolled almost eighteen million individuals, had developed working relationships with the body of physicians and hospitals, and was ready to pay for care. Seniors were hospitalized in institutions that were desegregated "overnight," rather than with "all deliberate speed."

Consider as well that President Johnson announced the War on Poverty in his State of the Union address in January, 1964 and that the Economic Opportunity Act was signed that very summer. Similarly, the Head Start initiative was developed during the winter of 1965 and by that same summer almost 600,000 children were enrolled in a program that proved so effective that by now it has served some 25 million children. We often underestimate how much can be accomplished and how quickly if we decide to do so. Even so, we should recognize that the very fact that Medicare and Head Start are often cited as programs that were implemented with remarkable speed is in itself a reminder that one should not assume they are the norm. Leadership qualities, fiscal impact, general acceptability, all these and more make a substantial difference. The selection of an appropriate timetable in the context of the political process that relies on legislation rather than executive order is one of the distinguishing characteristics of a master policy adviser.

Sometimes things move quickly; sometimes slowly. My colleague adopted new norms more rapidly if he was in the pool and less rapidly if he came from the locker room. Of course I wished he had shortened the process of change. Yet that did not diminish my awareness that he had changed and was continuing to change. Old habits and arrangements involving behavior and culture are not simple administrative matters. As we debate policy proposals at any organizational level in the provision of access to health care it is necessary to consider the often overlooked issue of timetables and phasing. It would be a pity indeed to move more slowly in enrolling the entire population and take longer than is necessary on the assumption that the political or administrative systems cannot move rapidly. It would, however, also be a tragedy to reject measured and coherent steps designed to build on one another on the grounds that they do not move us forward to the desired goal at a rapid enough pace. The history of many social policy proposals, including national health insurance, suggests the danger of rejecting measured and measurable progress while holding out for something bigger and better and faster. Regrettably, there is no general rule that tells us how quickly institutions can be changed, how rapidly behavior can be altered, what rate of speed is appropriate. Once again the policy adviser and the decision maker are forced to exercise their best judgment.

Is Everything Connected?

I have emphasized that policy advisers may find it advantageous and even necessary to redefine and sometimes broaden the policy issue they are asked to address. The "correct" definition of the problem is crucial. Nevertheless, even while many policies are interconnected, there are occasions when it is useful to "bite off small chunks" and to move forward even if only in a limited manner. Whether one picks up or loses allies by narrowing or broadening one's policy prescription will help determine how wide one casts the net and the choice of policy options one addresses.

One Sunday morning in the early 1970s I met with two Israeli health planners who worked in the Israel Ministry of Health and who were visiting—more correctly, taking a busman's holiday—in Boston. Years earlier both had attended graduate school in the United States, but they had not kept abreast of developments that were taking place or contemplated in American health policy. They had set up a series of appointments with members of the academic community who were involved in studying and teaching health management, policy, and planning. I had met with them at mid-week and we discussed subjects of mutual interest.

Since I had visited Israel numerous times and knew a fair amount about the Israeli health care system, I welcomed the opportunity to learn more about recent developments therein. They, in turn, learned more about the United States. Finding that they were still going to be in town over the weekend I offered to pick them up at their hotel on Sunday morning and walk around Harvard Square and Harvard Yard. Experience had taught me that though there were many interesting, beautiful, and historic venues in metropolitan Boston, Harvard environs were often the area that non-Bostonians were most interested in visiting.

And so it was that three of us were walking along Massachusetts Avenue past the Harvard Coop towards Church Street on our way to Harvard Yard. As we walked, we continued the conversation we had begun a few days earlier: the prospects for the enactment of some form of universal health insurance in the United States. Those prospects appeared bright in the early 1970s. Medicare had been enacted in 1965, implemented in 1966, and while health care expenditures had escalated and were viewed as a significant problem, the general consensus was that Medicare was a "building block," a "foundation stone," the first step toward universal coverage. President Nixon had proposed a Comprehensive Health Insurance Program (CHIP) and Representative Wilbur Mills and Senator Edward Kennedy had joined in offering an alternative that built upon the president's approach. There were a number of competing approaches toward assuring that a program would be universal in coverage, comprehensive in scope, efficient in its administration and in the delivery of medical care, and equitable in the way it was financed. The "experts" agreed that something would be enacted. The debate was not "whether," but "how."

There were those who wanted to extend the tax-based Medicare program so that it would cover the entire population. Others wanted to build upon the employer-employee health insurance link and expand employer insurance while providing subsidies to those firms and individuals unable to afford the insurance premiums. Still others argued for tax credits to individuals and like the negative income tax proposals then current presumed that checks would be issued to individuals whose tax payments were less than the credit would be. In somewhat similar fashion others favored a subsidized voucher system that would enable households to purchase health insurance policies. Some wanted to move rapidly to universality while others wanted to do so by phasing in different age groups over a period of time, perhaps beginning with children and working up to the Medicare age of sixty-five, perhaps starting with individuals just below sixty-five and working down to cover children. Many analysts expected a vigorous debate around the rich menu of proposals, as, in fact, ensued in the spring and summer of 1974. There was a good deal of optimism that the debate would not stall or derail enactment of some form of national health insurance. There seemed to be general agreement that we faced a problem that needed to be solved and that with compromise and good will Republicans and Democrats could fashion a solution. Few analysts would have believed that over thirty years later we would still be discussing the same problem and considering virtually the same and some additional options.

As I walked with my two colleagues, I was struck by the litter on the sidewalk. I had to kick aside the remains of Saturday night: the empty coke and beer cans, the cups which had held coffee or other liquids, the paper that had wrapped sandwiches, the cardboard pizza plates, the bags and other popcorn containers. It had been a normal Saturday night and I inferred that this was a "normal" Sunday morning.

I can still hear myself exploding. Picking up on the subject we had been discussing, I brought more than a bit of emotion and passion to the statement: "But we won't have national health insurance in the United States till Harvard Square is clean!" My Israeli colleagues stopped in surprise. Neither my statement nor the emotion with which it was delivered fit the analytic framework of our policy discussion. It was clear that I owed them (and, for that matter, myself) some sort of an explanation, some manner of matching and relating the content and tone to our more deliberative discourse.

The explanation that sufficed for that morning was the argument that a public that threw trash into a "collective common area" thereby gave evidence of an underdeveloped sense of community. Lacking that sense and set of values with which "community" was associated it would not press for a national health insurance program that included everyone and that shared costs in an equitable manner. All definitions of a universal health program necessarily involved some redistribution. In a tax-based program those with higher income would pay more to help support the health program than would those with lower income. In a private insurance based program individuals and households with lower income who otherwise could not afford the necessary premiums would be subsidized and the tax funds for the subsidy would, because of progressivity, be provided by others with higher income. One of the differences among the various proposals was that some were more explicit than others in recognizing that without redistribution one could not achieve universality.

I was going much further. I assumed redistribution had as a prerequisite a sense of community and I was using attitudes toward trash and trash disposal as a proxy for and definition of community.

Apparently I was prepared to argue that without that sense of community—as evidenced by a dirty Harvard Square—there would be insufficient support for national health insurance. I wanted to use private behavior, specifically about trash, toward the public common as a litmus test of attitudes toward NHI. One could not fail one part of the test without failing both parts. No compartmentalization for me!

My Israeli friends were kind. They heard me out, but decided not to pursue the subject. Perhaps they agreed with the general thrust, but surely they could have questioned why I singled out trash rather than free public libraries, free or virtually free higher education, adequately subsidized housing, and a myriad of other goods and services that would show a concern about one's neighbor. They chose not to press me for a more complete description of "community" and a more complete listing of the attributes I would include as part of a moral stance that adequately compensated for the disparities in the existing income distribution. Surely there was more to "community" than a clean Harvard Square. What would I add and where would I draw the line?

And they might have gone even further. They could have pointed out that a clean Harvard Square might not be how others might define "community." They might have argued that one could support universal health insurance for various reasons that had little to do with "justice" and "fairness" as I defined them. One might favor a universal program for efficiency reasons or, if constructed appropriately, as a cost containment or quality enhancement measure just as one might reject NHI because of the specter of "big government" even if one favored actions that in general would increase distributive justice. One's attitudes toward universal access to insurance and to health care may say a lot about an individual's value system as it applies to concern about others but, importantly, it may say very little. One's reaction to a piece of legislation that requires redistribution is not simply a matter of whether one feels empathy, but whether one believes the legislation would work and at what cost, if any, to other values one may hold, say, for example, principles of federalism or of privacy. The relationship I postulated was neither necessary nor sufficient. The policy adviser who responds to an inquiry about health insurance options with a "First we have to ask why folks throw sandwich wrappings on the sidewalk" has strayed too far in the redefinition of the question.

Some find it tempting to cast an argument in moral terms believing that their definition of ethical behavior is accepted by others and far more compelling than "mere" pragmatism. They would do well to remember that there are many ways to operationalize one's social conscience. The complexity and unpredictability, the inconsistency I see in others and the inconsistency they see in me cannot be assumed away. The various components of an index of cooperation, community, and "sharing" may "contradict" each other: one may donate money or time to food pantries even though one does not give up one's place in line or seat on the bus in order to assist someone who is elderly.

Today, some thirty years after my conversation with my Israeli colleagues, there once again is an increasing pressure for some sort of universal health program, but much of the support may have little to do with a feeling of empathy toward the over almost fifty million persons who are without insurance. By stressing the unhappy experiences of individuals with insurance rather than the problems of the uninsured, Michael Moore's movie *Sicko* rested its case for change in health financing arrangements largely on fear that what happened to others could happen to you, on self-interest rather than on empathy. Americans are concerned and frightened.

They are aware that though today they are insured they may lose their protections as firms cut back on insurance coverage and increase deductibles, co-insurance rates, and employee contribution in the face of increasing premium costs. They know that old-line manufacturing firms with large obligations both to their work force and retirees find it increasingly difficult to compete on price with newer firms with a younger work force and few retirees. They recognize that many of the uninsured receive care that is paid for by those with insurance and that such care is often more expensive than would have been the case had it been rendered in a different setting (the physician's office rather than the emergency room) or earlier (before the patient became sicker). They may favor a universal program on any of those grounds and believe that one can construct a program that would significantly reduce the very considerable administrative expenditures associated with today's private health insurance system. None of these factors rely on empathy or community. None rely on keeping Harvard Square clean.

It is true that various policy matters are connected and interconnected. Nevertheless they can be examined independently. The policy adviser may enjoy the spiritual "Dry Bones" (perhaps especially in the Fred Waring arrangement) that stresses connections:

> Your toe bone connected to your foot bone,
> Your foot bone connected to your ankle bone,
> Your ankle bone connected to your leg bone,
> Your leg bone connected to your knee bone,
> Your knee bone connected to your thigh bone,
> Your thigh bone connected to your hip bone,
> Your hip bone connected to your back bone,
> Your back bone connected to your shoulder bone,
> Your shoulder bone connected to your neck bone,
> Your neck bone connected to your head bone.

Nevertheless, enjoyable and educational as the policy analyst may find the song, a patient would not be well-served by a physician who was paralyzed by the complexity of these anatomical relationships when called upon to treat a hip fracture. So, too, if the policy adviser is so impressed by the way all policy matters interact with one another that he operates with an overriding belief that every question needs to be reformulated and broadened.

As has been pointed out, the effective policy adviser is an individual who is able to find the appropriate balance between competing and conflicting forces: principle and pragmatism, breadth and specificity, vision and political reality. In seeking balance, the adviser must be sensitive to issues of timing and the rate of change. Those who felt that President Johnson's call for a new way to think about and analyze government programs required too much change in too short a period of time were convinced that "you have to crawl before you walk." Their opponents who shared the same long term objectives were equally convinced that speed was essential, that if government agencies were permitted to crawl they'd be overcome with inertia. One might ask for so much change that, convinced that such change cannot be achieved in the relevant time period, one gives up and accomplishes nothing; one can ask for so little change that, convinced it won't make much of a difference, one relaxes and accomplishes nothing. America's call for less oil consumption and energy independence surely provides examples on both sides of the debate. The decision maker and her policy adviser who call for revolutionary change must recognize that revolutions do not occur in a slow, deliberate, and hesitant fashion. Daniel Burnham whose plans for Chicago were of great influence is often quoted as having stated, "Make no little plans. They have no magic to stir men's blood and probably will not themselves be realized." Neither, however, can great changes occur by advocating a program that seems so comprehensive and that would be implemented with such speed as to frighten potential allies away from the battle.

Is half a loaf better than none? Of course. But what if one had settled for only half when one might have obtained three-quarters of a loaf? What if, having received half a loaf, some allies drift away and, somewhat sated, abandon the battle for a full loaf—perhaps the enactment of Medicare and Medicaid reduced the pressure for a universal program? What if the energy sapped in getting half a loaf leaves one too weakened to fight for the other half? What if, by announcing in advance what one might settle for, one cannot even attain that compromise position? There are many, many "what ifs" in considering policy advice, strategy, and tactics. And they are answered not with a formula, but with judgment. The issues of the need to compromise and the art of reaching an accommodation pervade all fields of policy. It is certainly evident in health affairs where the battle is often joined between those who want to "go all the way," hoping that if they do not succeed they will have educated the electorate and in so doing increased the possibility that "it will be easier next time" and others who feel that small victories add up and may move one closer to the ultimate goal or failing that are "good" in their own right.

I testified at a Senate committee hearing in 1989 where just that issue arose. I had come a bit early and had the opportunity to greet Senator Edward Kennedy with whom I had worked on national health insurance matters for many years. He and I were each scheduled to testify on the broad issue of health insurance, but we were both aware that what each of us had to say would differ markedly. I, representing the Committee for National Health Insurance—which in the past had worked very closely with the senator—would be talking about the need to move with dispatch with legislation for universal coverage. While expressing a preference for something akin to a Medicare for All approach, I was prepared to accept and argue for a state by state approach with federal support for state initiatives, but only if whatever the mechanism the state selected covered its entire population and, thus, was truly universal. The senator was also ready to speak to the need for an expansion of available health insurance, but was prepared to focus on more proximate and more limited objectives that in his political judgment were attainable.

I had never looked forward to testifying before a Congressional committee. Though I had always been treated politely and in a friendly fashion my experience in watching the McCarthy hearings in the early 1950s and the way witnesses were badgered, harassed, assaulted, and insulted had made a lasting impression. I knew similar things would not happen to me, yet I accepted invitations to testify with great misgivings and only because I felt a sense of obligation to present the views that I believed in and thus strengthen the hand of others who shared those beliefs, convert some skeptics, or get one more idea onto the public agenda. Even so, when I received an invitation to testify I hoped that a schedule conflict would make it impossible for me to accept.

If that were true in general, it was especially so that day. I did not believe I would enjoy the session since my testimony would disagree with that of the senator whom I greatly respected. My task was not made easier by the comments made by the few colleagues who had accompanied me that the senator had abandoned the field of battle for national health insurance and, thereby, had weakened the "cause." They were angry that they had lost their most public ally and in their anger questioned his motives.

Not surprisingly, Senator Kennedy's testimony was compelling. It contained the right mix of "human interest" and of analytic backup. Moving between the particular Mrs. Jones and her difficulties and the millions of Mrs. Jones in the United States, he demonstrated that he would have been a superb physician/epidemiologist. As always, he knew his subject (not only his testimony) and knew how to convey both his pain at the situations he described and the fact that there were answers and solutions that could improve matters. Then, perhaps to convince those who he knew felt abandoned by what they viewed as his "compromises" and willingness to settle for "half a loaf" he turned and quite pointedly—I confess that I believed he was looking directly at me as he spoke—stated that there would be those who would argue that a Canadian-like system (the phrase "Medicare for All" had not yet achieved currency) would be more comprehensive, more efficient, and less costly and, as a consequence, more desirable and that he agreed that would be so. But that simply wasn't going to happen and he was not prepared to "hold hostage" those who could be helped today, those who would benefit from the legislation that he supported and that could be enacted. He was not prepared to force those who could be helped today to wait and wait and wait for more encompassing legislation. It was clear that he and I took different positions on how the agenda should be defined, the very kind of issue that bedevils those who deal with policy matters. Though troubled, I was able to leave the hearing room encouraged by the fact that my testimony in favor of "revolutionary" change helped cast Senator Kennedy as responsible and moderate.

I do not recount this brief story in order to lay the groundwork for assessing whether Senator Kennedy was right or wrong in his political evaluation that useful legislation could be enacted and that even with his support more encompassing and comprehensive legislation would fail. That evaluation is exceedingly complex. Perhaps support for comprehensive legislation would serve to educate other legislators and the public and thus hasten the day when it could be enacted. Perhaps limited legislation could not work effectively in the absence of more fundamental changes and if it didn't, that hurt the "cause." Perhaps what makes compromise possible is that there are those who press to go farther and faster. These, and similar questions, rely upon political judgment and Senator Kennedy's credentials far exceeded that of others engaged in this kind of debate. Even so, he could be in error. Nevertheless, it is not my purpose to evaluate and discuss the specific proposals he and I were presenting to the Senate Committee.

Rather, it is to stress that individuals with the same ultimate goal may differ markedly in their evaluation of the alternate paths to reach it and how long each of those paths might be. Earlier I suggested that an individual who supports a universal health insurance plan of what would be considered the most redistributive kind might, at the same time, throw litter from his car window or push his way to the front of a line. So I would also argue that an individual who supports a universal health insurance plan with liberal characteristics might, for pragmatic reasons, opt to move slowly and deliberately and in a limited way, though importantly in the right direction. To conclude that "high minded principle" should never yield to pragmatism may be a very considerable error. Indeed, it may even be one made for reasons that are self-serving: after all, it is easier to remain within the fraternity of like minded friends with whom one has fought "the good fight" than to "leave the reservation" and be criticized for abandoning one's principles.

The policy adviser, like all of us, is confronted by the need to make choices. In evaluating the choices that are made we must be careful not to adopt a posture of rigidity, one that assumes that if someone favors A one surely must also favor B, C, and D and that one should pick one's allies and designate one's opponents using that sort of template. Similarly, one should recognize that in human interaction, whether in the halls of Congress or at the kitchen table, the adoption of a philosophy that rules out compromise and that questions the motives and commitments of those who are "pragmatic" and do not believe that choices always involve "either-or" does not serve us well.

Once again, as in so many matters of public policy—and of life—there is a need for balance.

4

Knowing the "Other"

Learning from the Non-Expert

In the early 1960s I took a non-stop flight from Washington, D.C. to San Francisco. Since this was one of my first flights across the country, I spent much of the time looking out the window. I was astonished by the impressive and snow-capped Rockies, puzzled how it was that pioneers dared to embark across those mountains in covered wagons, and impressed by how large America is and by its ever changing terrain. I could not help but conclude that our nation's size and geographic differences would make for important differences in the experiences and attitudes of the people who lived under my flight path.

That America was a nation of differences was not a new insight. I had moved a lot by then. In addition to spending three years in Canada, I had lived in New York, Georgia, Pennsylvania, Connecticut, Maryland, the District of Columbia, and North Carolina. I had served in the United States Navy with shipmates whose backgrounds were very different—when some of them discovered I was Jewish they told me they had never met a Jew before and one was puzzled that I didn't have horns. I had followed presidential election results and was well aware of vastly different voting patterns. True, I had driven across the U.S., but the impact of seeing the nation unfold over a five-hour time period was very much greater than had been true over a trip that took five weeks. Indeed, the impact was so great that I concluded that high officials of our government, say secretaries and under-secretaries, should be required to travel across the country twice a year by air and be forced to look out the window—no memos, newspapers, or books—so they would be reminded how large and diverse our nation was. I thought that would be an important datum for policy makers.

But, valuable as such a reminder might be, it is far from sufficient. To know that there are differences does not inform us what those differences are and, therefore, does not tell us whether and to what degree they are germane to the implementation of a particular policy initiative. Nor does it increase our range of understanding and enable us to project with some degree of confidence whether and how particular policies might work or fail. We need to know much more than the fact that there are all kinds of Americans. The problem is that quite often the importance of the additional knowledge is ignored and that even when its need is recognized, it is not easily acquired. It must be consciously and deliberately sought out. Candidates who have campaigned for a party's nomination and then for the presidency, claim that doing so "broadened their horizons," but that opportunity is not open to all.

Decision makers and their advisers have few opportunities to hear "others" and quite often are so busy "doing" that they have little time for "listening." Most often they intersect only with persons who have essentially the same background, set of experiences, and attitudes as they. To some and perhaps an increasing degree that is true of all of us and may explain why after an election we so often hear expressions of surprise as we discover that there are a lot of folks who voted for another candidate: "Where did they come from? Everyone I know voted the way I did." Though we are all aware of the expression "inside the beltway" and its application to those who work for or intersect with government, the fact is that many individuals work inside their own beltway, that is, in a more homogeneous environment than is desirable. When that occurs they may lack vital information.

In the spring of 1969 there were rumors that Boston's proposed Brigham and Women's Hospital would soon begin construction of its new, expanded, and much needed medical center. This new facility, adjacent to Harvard Medical School, would be the final step in the merger of three existing Harvard affiliated hospitals: the Peter Bent Brigham, the Robert Breck Brigham, and the Boston

Hospital for Women. That all three institutions, housed in old and surely technologically outdated buildings, needed these upgraded facilities was beyond dispute. When I visited my sister-in-law after the birth of my niece in the Boston Lying-In Hospital—which together with the Free Hospital for Women formed the Boston Hospital for Women—the dust, dirt, and grime on and in the screens on the windows of her room seemed and may have been as old as the hospital itself. While this did not reflect on the quality of medical care available to patients, it was both frustrating and more than disconcerting to all who practiced in or used the institution. Nevertheless, though there was agreement about the need for new facilities, there was considerable tension about the plans for the hospital.

At least in part this was due to the history of the site that the new institution was to occupy. Planning for the merger of the three institutions had begun much earlier. Indeed, in earliest discussions, the merger would have included Children's Hospital—but things moved so slowly and Children's needs were so great that that institution proceeded to "go its own way." The remaining three institutions approached Harvard Medical School and urged that, since the school had a sufficiently large endowment, it purchase the triple-decker houses that lined the side of Francis Street opposite the existing Peter Bent Brigham, a long, low structure that stretched for what seemed like miles. The proposal was that when the hospitals were ready and had acquired the necessary funds the houses would be torn down and on their site the new hospital would be built.

The existing Brigham was an institution in which one met colleagues by walking the long hall. Indeed, the distinguished chief physician, George Thorn told me that staff knew that he would walk the hall—make his rounds as it were—twice a day and looked forward to the opportunity to meet him without being required to make an appointment. The culture of a horizontal building like the Brigham was vastly different than that of a vertical building with a bank of elevators rather than a long corridor, as, for example, was the case in the Massachusetts General Hospital. In vertical buildings if people meet, they do so in elevators and by accident;

they do not wander halls on floors except, perhaps, the one they work on. "Cross fertilization" is, therefore, more readily achieved in horizontal buildings. Though there was no final design for the new "Brigham and Women's Hospital," the Francis Street owner occupied and rental properties met all locational requirements and, given the number of city blocks available, would not require "skyscraper" construction.

Harvard purchased the houses in order to hold them for the "appointed day" when the hospitals would officially merge and, having prepared their plans, would be ready to build. It did not evaluate this "investment" on the basis of the rate of return; its motives were quite different. Though many if not most of the property owners left when they sold, the triple deckers remained occupied with former and new tenants. Harvard anticipated a relatively quick "turn around" and saw no need to raise rents during this anticipated short term. As it turned out, however, the process was exceedingly slow. As the years passed the difference between market rents and the rents being charged by Harvard grew. By 1968 tenants were paying substantially less than they would have had to pay for similar rental properties in Boston. On the other hand, the units were in a state of minor disrepair. Because the construction of the new hospital on the very site occupied by the houses was always "just around the corner," very little was spent on maintenance and upkeep of the units.

Then quite unexpectedly, in the winter of 1968-1969 there was an announcement that the hospitals had developed an architectural plan for the new institution and that construction would soon begin. Inevitably, therefore, there was considerable tension to be found among those who lived in the triple story, three family buildings. It was not only that they liked their neighborhood, but also that they were aware of, and frightened by, the very severe budget issues they would confront when they entered the Boston housing market. In addition to having to pay moving expenses they would face very substantial increases in the sums they would have to allocate for rent. While analysts could point to the "bargain" the residents had been getting—even adjusted for the quality of housing—that did not solve the budget problem the displaced individuals and families would face.

Francis Street and its tensions were one short block from Harvard Medical School and in April 1969 Harvard, like many if not most American colleges and universities, experienced its own tensions in large measure related to the war in Vietnam, the bombing of Cambodia, and a general distrust of what was viewed as an "establishment" that was complicit in all that was going wrong. The institution also faced stresses associated with what were seen as "encroachments" by Harvard on Cambridge and Boston neighborhoods and communities. Certainly of greatest importance in building tensions, were events stemming from the night of April 10 when a number of students occupied an administration building in Harvard Yard and Nathan Pusey, the president of the University, called in the police who, using force, expelled the students. In turn, this galvanized the larger community of students who, though uninvolved in the takeover, protested the actions by the president and by the state and Cambridge police. Each problem—the Harvard Yard "bust," the housing issues near the medical school, the references to plans not made public for the new hospital—interacted with the others and grew.

In earlier years it would probably have been the case that Harvard and its affiliated hospitals could have, and would have, gone ahead with their construction plans while ignoring whatever grumbling the persons about to be displaced or otherwise negatively affected might have voiced. But by the spring of 1969 it was no longer an accepted dictum that sections of a city could be razed with little regard for residents, neighborhood, and community and be replaced by new construction that would automatically be defined as "progress." Nor was it an accepted dictum that "experts" were expert; Vietnam had put that concept to rest. And it certainly was no longer the case that large institutions could assume that they could easily ignore and outwait a bit of complaining, a few letters to the editor, and similar decorously expressed "differences of opinion"—one could hardly call them "protests." Even the Kennedy Presidential Library whose planned location was next door to Harvard was forced to find a different location!

Whatever the physicians, nurses, educators, managers, and employees thought about "ownership" of the Brigham and Women's, the people who would use the hospital believed that in a very real sense it belonged to them. The combination of general community involvement, resident concern, and student protest finally led to a public meeting in one of the Medical School amphitheatres. The meeting was designed to provide an opportunity for the leaders of the Brigham and Women's Hospital to present the "vision" and the plans for the new facility as well as the process and the timetable that would be followed to translate the plans into reality. It would also provide an opportunity for the various attendees to voice their comments and concerns. I am certain that the hospital officials who were the presenters were convinced that once their plans were explained and the benefits of the new facility made clear, all attendees—even including those who lived in the triple-deckers on Francis Street—would withdraw whatever reservations they might have had and voice their endorsement.

I knew the medical and lay leaders—all men—who would speak and was aware that humility and wishy-washy convictions were not their strong suits. In general, they were persons who held and were prepared to voice strong opinions and who were—appropriately—proud of their achievements and the achievements and accomplishments of Harvard and its affiliated hospitals, the institutions with which they were associated. These were men whose long association with premier institutions had led to a kind of arrogance that encouraged them to believe that their views were necessarily correct and puzzlement that others did not recognize that was the case.

Thus, at a meeting at which a resident of one of the houses on Francis Street was berating the gracious, self-effacing, and mild mannered dean of the Harvard Medical School, Robert Ebert, and criticizing him in extremely personal terms, the chairman of the board of the Peter Bent Brigham walked over and in a shocked tone, implying that an apology was necessary, said, "Do you know to whom you are speaking? That's the *dean of the Harvard Medical School!*" He did not understand how it could be that, instead of an expression of contrition, he received a "so what's the big deal" response.

The evening of the community meeting the auditorium was packed with persons who were just curious, residents of the blocks near the hospital, students who were sympathetic to the residents' concerns or simply anti-establishment, faculty, and hospital as well as medical school administrators and employees. Also in attendance were the members of the community relations committee that the dean had formed shortly after the "bust" in Harvard Yard when students at the medical and dental schools joined the general student protest even though the Harvard medical and dental schools were located in Boston and geographically, as well as in other respects, distant from the center of the university in Cambridge. Indeed, these students went out on "strike" and presented the dean with a list of "demands" many of which were related to the housing issues that would result from the implementation of the plans for the newly merged hospital. In response, the dean established a committee of faculty, employees, administrators, and students to explore the housing problems that would arise when plans for hospital construction moved forward and to recommend policies to address those issues. Subsequently, when—at the request of the chairman and with the help of members of Students for a Democratic Society (SDS)—the affected residents were organized into a community organization with a leadership that could be part of a negotiation process, they also joined the committee.

The major presentation at the well-attended meeting was made by the distinguished surgeon in chief of the Peter Brent Brigham, Dr. Francis Moore. He was a person respected by all in the medical community, an individual whose picture had appeared on the cover of *Time* magazine some five years earlier and who was featured in its lengthy article on important advances in surgery. He spoke in a somewhat imperious and aloof manner conveying a sense of authority. When he concluded, he asked for comments and questions. One individual, a dark-skinned African-American whose physical attributes and demeanor, though not those of a Brahmin, also conveyed power and authority rose to his feet. Mel King, some fifteen years younger than Dr. Moore and certainly not part of the "establishment," had his own sizeable constituency. A former mathematics teacher, he had become a community organizer and an individual who was already making his mark on Boston and on

Boston politics. Undoubtedly he knew who Dr. Moore was; it is not likely that Dr. Moore knew who Mel King was.

Their "conversation" went something like this:

"You're not going to build that hospital. Not that way, Doc."

"Really? Why?"

"Because you haven't talked to us."

"Who are you? What do you know about the design of hospitals?"

"Doc., we are the patients and the families of patients. We know. We spend more time in those hospital rooms than you and the other doctors who wander in do."

Whatever the rest of the conversation, whatever the questions and answers, it was clear that there was more than a "communications problem." The "experts," the men with long experience, certainly could not and did not understand that there were things they might learn from non-experts. Indeed, as I discovered many years later, the Brigham's senior physicians had not felt it necessary to consider seriously the views of the medical residents who had important misgivings about the design and layout of the new hospital within which they would work. Of course, the meeting and the discourse were overlaid by a history of an "elitist" Harvard and of the Brigham which was viewed as a bad neighbor, an institution that had not established or affiliated with a single neighborhood or community health center, that looked inward rather than outward, and that had not really related to those individuals who were its closest neighbors, including those who lived across the street or in the adjoining public housing project.

Some of these characteristics were not at all different than those found in the relationships between many teaching hospitals and their surrounding community since historically such hospitals had been built in neighborhoods populated by low income individuals and persons of color who would be "teaching material" for medical students. Perhaps some of the speakers at the evening meeting shared the attitudes of a former leader of the Johns Hopkins medical community who had publicly lamented the spread of Blue Cross hospital insurance because "if everyone became a private instead of a ward patient, who would be left as teaching material?"

Thus, that evening meeting in a medical school amphitheatre—a bit of "enemy" territory—included complexities of race and economic and social status as well as the specific problem of the individuals who would be displaced by the new construction. They were a special case within what could be considered the broader mix of urban redevelopment and the civil rights revolution of the 1960s. Even so, I believe that the tensions at that meeting related in largest measure to the clash between the experts who presumably knew everything there was to know about building a hospital and the "little" people. Carl Sandburg's "The People, Yes" was not part of the meeting's agenda or perspective.

And so it was that I went up to Dr. Moore after the meeting. I knew him well for he served on the community relations committee which I chaired. I asked him whether the home he lived in had been designed by an architect and if so, whether there had been an occasion when he or his wife had turned to one another and said something like: "Why? Why did that architect have the door open to the right when he could so easily have hung it so it opened to the left where it wouldn't block the person getting a coat from the hallway closet from exiting the front door?" I asked whether there were times when they wondered why things were done in a manner that turned out to be inconvenient or that did not meet their needs. The answer, given with great feeling, was that indeed there were a number of such cases and that many of them could and should have been anticipated.

That was the response I had expected and I, therefore, tried to suggest that was what the very same issue that Mel King was talking about. I did not amplify the point; it seemed self evident. I turned out to have been far too delicate. I was so subtle that my question and comment had no impact. Perhaps my problem was that I could not cite the specific complaints that Mel King might have had in mind. Certainly it was the case that the inadequacies of the physical layout that I became acquainted with many years later when I was a parent of a hospitalized patient were unknown to me at that time. It is of interest that in largest measure those inadequacies in fact related to matters that raised problems for patients and family members, the very things that Mel King was referring to and that senior physicians had overlooked or, if aware, had seen as matters of low priority. Nevertheless, I believe the fundamental problem did not relate to issues of specificity, but to the more common failure to appreciate what non-experts might know and to see things from their vantage point.

I do not discount the knowledge that experts bring to bear on problems. The issue, once again, is one of balance. Most persons are not experts, but have gained knowledge and understanding through experience. Often they recognize issues that are unknown to the practitioners or experts or appreciate matters to which practitioners are simply not sensitive. All of us live with limited and compartmentalized knowledge. Dr. Moore could not see the similarity between his layman's experiences with architects and the patient's experiences with hospital designers. But the issue raised is quite a common one: the failure or inability to generalize, to understand that others, including persons with far less "training" but with personal experience, can see things that experts—and that, of course, includes those deeply involved with policy matters—cannot discern.

This issue, though found in many areas of endeavor, has been especially evident in the case of medicine. Historically, patients had been intimidated by physicians and had reacted in a generally docile manner. If they complained, it was to their friends or relatives, but not to the physician. Doctors were privy to the experts' knowledge and experience and the patient was the unequal dependent. The physician's white coat trumped the hospital johnny. It is only recently that physicians have learned that they dare not assume that their judgments and priorities are the same ones held by patients, that decisions on matters of treatment—for example, surgery or other interventions, hip replacement or "making do"—should reflect patient preferences not physician values, attitudes, or guesses about what the patient should or would prefer. Indeed, they cannot assume that because they have been sick or hospitalized they know what it is to be sick or hospitalized. I have heard physicians try to make that case, but what they ignore is that even as they lie in the hospital bed, they have a fund of knowledge that most of us who are non-physicians lack and that while they may fear the known, the rest of us fear both the known and the unknown.

It is true that medicine is changing. Yet, the general problem remains: the inability to comprehend fully that people on different sides of the desk or table have unequal knowledge, power, and priorities, therby increasing the likelihood that the professional can be unaware of or forget to consider the tastes and needs, experience and insights of the other. The issues raised may be dismissed as a "communications problem" with almost an implied suggestion that the word "mere" or "simple" should precede "communications problem." But that is to treat the matter far too lightly. Effective policies and appropriate decisions that affect people are far less likely to be developed in the absence of a commitment to listen and to learn from the attitudes and experience of all affected parties. That is as true for the policy adviser whether in government or elsewhere as it is the case in medicine.

I was present at a medical school faculty council meeting when a very able medical student was speaking about the benefits of the hand-held mini-computer he carried with him as he made rounds. It enabled him to call up all sorts of medical information that might aid him in his diagnoses and he could enter all sorts of patient information that he gathered as he stood at the foot of the patient's bed and asked the set of relevant questions. He was pleased that he did not have to rely on his memory to write things down when he left the room; he could enter it in "real time." The keyboard on the device necessarily was very small and thus the various keys were cramped together. And so I could not help but ask whether he could type his notes without looking at the keys. The answer was a quick and clear "no." I was distressed for I remembered carrying on a conversation with a physician who was looking at his computer screen even as we conversed. I could not help but feel that I was not receiving his full attention. I realized that the need to take notes on the mini-computer meant that this student no longer made eye contact with the patient. In doing so, he may have appeared uninterested, distant, and aloof and may have left the patient dissatisfied. As a consequence, he also may have denied himself valuable information: perhaps the patient's visual reaction to the questions, perhaps additional comments that might have been offered to a "friendlier" and more engaged physician, information might have benefitted the patient.

I tell that story not because I believe all patients are alike and would react as I. Patients differ and one must remember and apply the principle my mother articulated: "Some people like chicken and some people don't." I tell it in order to remind ourselves that all of us, whatever our expertise, be we attorney or architect, carpenter or cleaner, politician or physician, needs to learn how his or her expert judgment must be modified to incorporate the knowledge that persons with a different set of experiences bring to the table. Whether one is designing a hospital or structuring the encounter with a patient, it is important to learn from others what they deem important.

Experience Counts

The prescription I advocate is not unique to the medical arena. It is an ancient prescription about much broader issues. It can be found in the motto of the Southeastern Correctional Ministry, taken from the New Testament, Hebrews 13:3 "Remember those in prison as if you were their fellow prisoners, and those who are mistreated as if you yourselves were suffering." As well, it is found in the Passover Haggadah where one is reminded that in Exodus it is written that "In each generation, each person should feel as though he or she had gone forth from Egypt" and "You shall not oppress a stranger, for you know the feeling of a stranger having been strangers in the land of Egypt." Similarly, the approach is related to an op-ed piece by Douglas MacKinnon, one-time press secretary to Senator Bob Dole and a former White House and Pentagon official. It appeared in the New York Times on May 21, 2002.[1]

Mr. MacKinnon's op-ed piece was entitled "The Welfare Washington Doesn't Know." It began: "As Congress considers how to improve welfare reform, its members should understand what anyone with an ounce of common sense already knows: Most welfare recipients who left or were knocked off the welfare rolls are still struggling to survive. Within the Republican Party, I find myself in a tiny minority as a white male who grew up on welfare and was homeless on a number of occasions. For people who have not lived through these experiences and for far too many lawmakers, welfare recipients are nothing more than statistics or the subject of abstract policy debates. Few politicians in a position to affect people—positively or negatively—who are living below the poverty line have themselves ever come close to that line. *But to craft sound legislation, they have to have a real understanding of how that America lives* [my italics]." That last sentence bears repeating. It is that understanding of the "other" that assists us in viewing matters from a different vantage point and that is necessary in the crafting of policy.

By the time he was seventeen, Mr. Mackinnon and his family had been evicted thirty-four times. He writes of the "shame and pain" when "officers come to throw you out of your home and pile all your worldly possessions on the sidewalk for passerby to see." He echoes Hebrews and the Haggadah when he states "politicians who want to understand [the poor], (a horrifying $14,630 for a family of three) should imagine themselves counting and rolling pennies to buy food, medicine, or a subway fare." So it is that one can tie together Hebrews, Exodus, and Douglas Mackinnon, designing a hospital, and creating a situation in which one can learn from a patient. They all involve something greater than analyzing data: the desire and ability to listen to the "other" and thus becoming better able to imagine what it is like to be that other. These are prerequisites to the design of effective policies that affect individuals.

There are occasions when we learn that experience can take many forms. The physician who has practiced and listened to his or her patients may possess information that is denied to others even including specialists who know the data, but who have a limited range of experience on the ground. The same phenomenon may occur with the policy maker or adviser. The legislator who returns to the home district for a "town hall" meeting is likely to learn more than is gained from the local newspaper. The policy adviser who relies only on "experts," perhaps is destined to become an expert, but is unlikely to become a valued and valuable adviser.

Experience counts. Some years ago I was diagnosed as having something that I understood was akin to an adult version of infectious mononucleosis. I had gone to my physician with a low grade fever and with very little energy. I might have just "waited it out," but had an out-of-town lecture scheduled and could sense that as things were developing I would not have the desire or stamina to fulfill my commitment. So, like millions of my fellow citizens, I looked to American medicine to take care of and solve my problem. After examination and the appropriate tests I was given the diagnosis and was told to forget about the lecture, go home, take it easy, and come back for further tests in about a week.

I had no difficulty in "taking it easy;" I had no energy to do otherwise. I also discovered that I had no capacity for maintaining any activity requiring a significant span of attention. Daytime television—soaps since it was before *Law and Order*—was not of interest, I didn't seem to be up to serious reading, and discovered that even mystery stories could not engage me. I was forced to watch our local public broadcast station's coverage of the Massachusetts legislature, drifting off periodically, and then trying to discern whether I had really missed anything other than a quorum call.

I returned a week later for further blood tests and was sent home once again with the same advice to relax and take it easy. This pattern continued for some weeks. Perhaps I was feeling a bit better, but it was clear that I was not yet well. And so I kept going back to my physician for the periodic tests and update. On one such occasion, as I was coming out the door of our apartment building, I bumped into a neighbor coming in. He was a relatively young physician specializing in infectious disease and with an appointment in one of Boston's three medical schools. I knew that he was well regarded by colleagues.

"What are you doing home in the middle of the day?" he asked. I told him that I was headed out to see my internist and that I had this "adult version of mono," whose name I surely knew at the time, but have long since forgotten. "Ah, and what are you doing for it?" he inquired. I responded, "Nothing, really. I'm just staying home and doing as I was told, taking it easy." He looked at me and shook his head: "There's not a single study, not a single article in the *New England Journal of Medicine* that provides any evidence that taking it easy makes any difference at all in outcome. Your problem will simply run its course and one day you'll wake up feeling better. In the meantime you can go to work and resume your normal activities. You will not delay or in any other way affect your recovery."

I thanked him, got in the car and went to my physician. After some hesitation I shared this unsolicited "second opinion" with him. He responded quite quickly that my infectious disease friend who practiced in the medical school's hospital was quite correct in stating that there had not been a study of the matter. He, too, did not believe that the *NEJM* or the *Journal of the American Medical Association* (*JAMA*) had published any article on the appropriate treatment of the condition and, certainly, not on the efficacy of non-intervention and of taking it easy. But then he added an additional perspective. He suggested that my friend practiced in the hospital and most probably had little contact with patients with my condition. Furthermore, he did not have the opportunity to follow patients over an extended period of time. He saw them as in-patients, discharged them when it seemed appropriate—length of stays, it is true, were much longer in those days thus making for more patient-physician contact than would be the case today—and might or might not see them again on a follow up visit. He may well not have known how the patient fared after he or she left the hospital, unless things took a turn for the worse.

My internist suggested that since, in contrast, he had an office-based practice he did see patients—just as he was seeing me—over a span of some weeks. Albeit there were no articles suggesting he was correct, his experience was that taking it easy appeared to have beneficial effects and no harmful side-effects. In any case, it seemed to fit the patient's lack of energy and, thus, both the inability and lack of desire to do more. "What's wrong with taking it easy, especially if that's what you feel like doing?" was his final observation.

I found the last point compelling. Nevertheless, I also believed that the earlier observations about reliance on published research and on experience also seemed to have merit. Thus the issue of the weight to place on experience as compared with well designed research studies, perhaps even the question of the art versus the science of medicine was raised. On one side stood the academic researcher/practitioner whose knowledge base was heavily dependent on published studies. Absent the studies that would recommend specific interventions, the recommendation seemed to be to continue normal activities. On the other side stood the physician who, because of the nature of his practice and his years of experience, had encountered more patients with the specific condition. Absent the studies, he felt quite comfortable in relying on his experience to guide his actions.

I recognize that resolving the difference I sketch seems easy. Experience trumps ignorance—if we define ignorance as the absence of research studies—and even more so when experience suggested a rather "comfortable" therapy. It's certainly not hard to conclude that experience trumps "evidence based" medicine when, in fact, there is no evidence. Yet, as I thought about the problem, presumably while taking it easy, I found that it raised questions that were not easily resolved. On the one hand we might expect that the well designed research study would provide more generalizable and more rigorous findings than one physician's experiences, especially since—absent a research methodology—experiences tend to be impressionistic and, perhaps, heavily influenced by the most recent cases. On the other hand individual patients are individuals who share many characteristics in common, but who also exhibit important differences. Each patient is a reminder of inevitable variation. Five-year survival rates are not 100 percent or 0 percent. They lie somewhere in between. Some patients "make it" and others don't and what we want and need to know is the explanation for this phenomenon. Differences do matter and the ability to sense and be sensitive to those differences may come out of experience.

One can sympathize with physicians and policy analysts who value experience and consider it an important input into their decisions. The physician may feel that his or her experience is vitally important and that the ability to call upon it is what defines the word "professional" and distinguishes it from the term "technician." Mackinnon's words make clear his view that knowing the attitudes and experiences of others is vital to wise and informed policy. Yet in a world that seems increasingly dominated by data and by protocols, the value of qualitative information is often discounted and experience is often considered as the antithesis of science. This point was driven home to me in the cafeteria of Boston's Beth Israel Hospital when my father was an in-patient.

I had come to the hospital early on a weekend morning, had gone up to my father's room, found that he was sleeping, and repaired to the cafeteria for a cup of coffee. As I walked away from the cashier I saw a colleague, a vascular surgeon, sitting alone at a table sipping his coffee. I knew him since we served on a committee together and went over to sit with him. I greeted him asking him how things were going. Instead of the usual "fine," "OK," or "not too bad" I was told things were rotten. I asked what was wrong and discovered that my colleague was more than willing to pour out his anger and frustration. Perhaps it was simply that I was there, had asked, and that he needed to vent; perhaps it was that he knew I was a social scientist who studied health care organization and financing and he recognized that I would be interested in his tale of woe. More than likely it was a bit of both.

He was correct: I was quite interested and the more so since he was a valued colleague. It seems that some days earlier he was to perform a complex surgical procedure on a frail patient who lived some considerable distance from Boston. Given the rather long and arduous trip and the patient's state of health, my colleague wanted him to be admitted to the hospital two days before surgery in order to have the time to assure that the patient was stable. My colleague knew that admitting the patient that early was outside the ever more and more shortened norm—I remember the anger of an operating room nurse who was used to and believed in a more relaxed schedule when she informed me that under a new hospital policy patients who were to undergo open heart surgery were admitted in the morning for surgery in the afternoon.

Concerned that the patient's insurance carrier might refuse payment for the extra days in hospital, the physician attempted to get preadmission approval. As he described it, he was on the phone with multiple calls for the better part of a day and a half "talking with some twenty-year-old youngster who was staring at a computer screen in some central office in mid-America and telling me that the procedure that I was about to do did not require the extra hospitalization. It wasn't part of the protocol and she wouldn't approve it." It took a day plus of arguing, appealing, going up the line to supervisory personnel (and perhaps proving that he had not made a similar request in the past) till he finally received approval.

It was clear that one of the things that angered my colleague was the time that he had to spend on the matter. Yet it seemed to me that he was also angered, and perhaps to an even greater extent, by the insult: the fact that "the twenty-year-old youngster" who knew no medicine but could read a computer screen could negate the validity of his years of surgical experience. His professional judgment was questioned and ignored and with that his professionalism.

His story is not unique. Countless physicians have been affected by similar situations. They may feel that a diagnostic test or procedure is warranted, but that the insurance carrier might not approve; they may feel that another day of hospital observation is appropriate, but that the predetermined reimbursement associated with the particular diagnosis would mean that the extra day would hurt the institution's bottom line. They have been accustomed to calling for more resources, not for less. They resent the intrusion of others—most especially, of non-MDs—into their exercise of clinical judgments. They may understand that a nation that is searching for ways to slow down the growth in medical expenditures and that is increasingly aware that wide variations in physician behavior and resource utilization appear unrelated to outcomes, would focus its attention on influencing and even on controlling physician behavior. Yet, it is not hard to understand that the individual physician hardly views her or his behavior as profligate and is angered by what is perceived as a new ethos in which economics rules the roost. Under such conditions—when experience hardly counts—tension and conflict are the inevitable byproducts.

The story of such conflicts between experience and protocols, between looking for the variation and relying on the averages, is not found only in medicine. The classroom teacher and the principal who have succeeded in defying predictions about the performance of their students and their school may know what they are doing "right" and be well aware that that may not be following the template developed by and called for by the school district. Nevertheless it may be difficult to convince others of the validity of the "on the ground" decisions they made. A *Washington Post* article back in the 1960s told about a school in the District of Columbia whose students performed in a manner that defied all expectations. In spite of the enrollment of mostly disadvantaged children in an old and more than likely understaffed school with few resources, reading skills were far higher than expected and exceeded the city average for the various grade levels. The article suggested that the explanation lay in the fact that the staff was comfortable with whatever reading material the youngsters used in honing their skills—and that included comic books. Personnel had made a decision that the important thing was that the children read rather than what they read. Performance increased because experienced teachers had the confidence to step outside the boundaries set by higher authorities. Parents who have watched their children calculate batting averages and have noticed that their offspring understand why it is much easier to raise an average at the beginning of the season than at the end appreciate that one can learn a lot of mathematic concepts from what many would consider frivolous: the sports pages.

In medicine there is a need for an appropriate balance between the economic pressures not to "waste" resources, the appropriate reliance on the science of medicine and its epidemiological base, and the ability to call upon experience to reach judgments about the individual patient. Regrettably, there is abundant evidence that we have not yet achieved that balance. Part of the problem may be that the policy maker can not easily adjudicate among each of the actors in the drama. That, unfortunately, will leave my surgeon colleague unhappy and insulted and the gatekeeper who must deal with pre-admission and other clinical intervention approvals harassed and angry. One hesitates to consider where this all leaves the confused patient.

Regrettably, there is no formula by which to learn how to identify with the evicted child, the patient, the prisoner, the slave, and the downtrodden. Some college presidents, journalists, and commentators have spent months and longer working at the menial jobs that many Americans fill, the better to understand the hard life that many Americans live. But most of us will have to learn about the other America in other ways. And, in a sense, that is true of even our college presidents and journalists and commentators, who, after all, were very much aware that their condition was only temporary, that they could leave at any time and, in fact, would soon depart. So how do we and the policy analyst learn what it is to be poor, what it is to be ill and without health insurance, what it is to be the other?

One way is to listen; another is to read. I have little question that many of us have insights into the impact of 9/11 on those in or near the World Trade towers because we read the day after day after day short obituaries in the *New York Times* as well as the various accounts of pain and hurt and anguish and heroism and of triumph. Quite often that kind of writing is done by journalists who know how to listen and how to tell a human-interest story that puts faces on the statistics and tell us what the otherwise dry statistics really represent, that as a colleague put it: "Statistics are human beings with the tears wiped dry."

Some years ago a reporter for a weekly news magazine came to my office to interview me. Having listened to my telling him about the number of persons without any or with inadequate health insurance, he expressed some doubt about the data and wondered where the uninsured I spoke about really were, telling me: "All my friends have health insurance." I sent him across the street to the shoemaker, pizza parlor, greasy spoon, and local Arby's and told him to ask the people behind the counters about their insurance coverage. He listened to them and returned shaken. These owners or employees of very small and, at best, marginally successful businesses had no insurance coverage and couldn't afford it. They were gambling on their good health and were frightened that they might lose that gamble. Perhaps, just perhaps, listening enabled him to begin to understand and see things he had not seen before.

Unless one is, one doesn't really know what it is to be an African-American in the United States, or a Latino, disabled or poor, uninsured or otherwise disadvantaged. For that matter, most of us do not and will not know what it is to be really wealthy. That is not knowledge acquired by thinking about it. We—that, of course, includes those who advise on matters of policy—have to want to know and have to start with a knowledge base acquired by reading and listening.

Advisers in the health policy domain and those who administer health programs, need to become much better acquainted with the patient's and the physician's perspective. They and all of us need to consider the arguments made by those who differ with our views and, importantly, consider how it is that they find those arguments believable and appropriate. It is not that in doing so we would learn how to present our approaches more effectively and convincingly, although that might occur. Rather, it is because we might gain insights that would help us enrich, refine, and improve our own proposals.

We All Play Many Roles

Sometimes, through circumstance, we are cast in multiple roles and unexpectedly discover the difference in outlook that each role entails. We are forced to realize that being "we" is not enough, that we also must consider that which we learn when we become "others." Needless to say, it is an illuminating experience. We are forced to recognize that the perspective each role entails has value and that the several perspectives must be reconciled.

The matter I refer to is illustrated by an incident that took place almost twenty years ago. At that time, I had a wonderful, an exemplary, physician. Fifty years ago he would have been described—in a term that is not used as frequently today—as a superb "diagnostician." He kept up with the literature and had the opportunity to discuss the latest therapies and drugs when he intersected with young medical students and residents at the bedside of a hospitalized patient. It was a time, not often found in today's world, when non-hospital based physicians were not hard pressed and, thus, were able to visit their hospitalized patients whose hospital stays were long enough for students, residents, and the attending physician to meet over a period of days. My physician learned from those who knew the most recent research results; in turn he shared the knowledge that can be gained only over a period of time, the knowledge based on experience.

He was of the "old school." He entered medicine in an earlier period, when physicians had the time to engage in conversation with and exhibit concern for the patient. His patient appointments were for thirty minutes—sometimes they took a bit longer, sometimes a bit less. I never left his office with an unasked or unanswered question. He never signaled that our encounter was over by writing a prescription, handing it to me, standing up, and walking me to the door. I certainly was not aware of a glance to the wrist watch.

Examinations began with a conversation about any new developments in my medical and general life and a review of any recent developments related to symptoms and, as I grew older, aches and pains that I had mentioned at the previous visit and which, since he was older, he assured me he also had. Only when that discussion was concluded was I told to go into the examination room, disrobe, and wait for him to appear. That happened in a few minutes since with only one examination room he did not schedule more than one patient at a time. After the examination he went into his office, wrote up the chart while I dressed, and waited for me to join him for a conversation about his findings and their implications.

It was all very different from a physician encounter I had many years earlier when I was a graduate student. I had a pain in my ear and my doctor, a general practitioner, examined me, told me that I had a fungus infection in my ear and referred me to a specialist who would "get rid of it." For some reason—perhaps a word was used that led me astray—I assumed that the fungus would be "scraped out" and I envisioned an extremely painful procedure. I went to the specialist who placed what I believe was a long narrow electric bulb in my ear, turned a switch, and almost immediately told me that we were through and that I should make an appointment for a week hence. He did not mention the diagnosis; he did not tell me what he had done or intended to do. The only real communication was that I would need another appointment in a week. I said that I would make that arrangement and added that while I recognized that a physician cannot predict the course of events with certainty I hoped he could tell me whether I would be coming in once a week for an extended period of time, perhaps even a year; whether this was a matter of months; or whether it would require only a few visits. I know that I asked all that with extreme diffidence for at that time that was viewed as the appropriate patient-physician relationship. His reply to my question was stunning: "If you wanted to know that, why didn't you go to medical school?" Even in 1950 when physicians did not think it necessary to share information with the patient and when "expert" physicians made decisions on behalf of "dependent" patients the crude response was more than three standard deviations from the norm.

By the latter part of the century the relationship between physicians and patients had changed. The norm had altered. We were entering into the age of "consumerism," a time in which patients dared to ask questions, request second opinions, and share in medical decision making. Some patients didn't adjust easily: my father felt that asking for a second opinion was an insult to his doctor and would jeopardize their relationship; some physicians didn't adjust easily: they were used to and enjoyed commanding the ship. Nevertheless, medicine is not immune to the pressures of social forces in the greater society. As part of a culture in which the role of the expert was being redefined, medicine, too, changed.

Yet, the physician whom I earlier described as "exemplary" had no adjustment problem. He practiced as he had practiced, sharing information and continuing to exhibit unusually friendly, solicitous behavior. He, too, was three standard deviations from the norm—but in a positive direction. His problem was not with patients whose demands were changing—his patient panel was older and probably more fixed in their ways—but with the medical care reimbursement and payment system that questioned the "excessive" time he spent with patients, the number of tests he called for, the dollar implications of his medical decisions. For a time he succeeded in dealing with patients without being constrained by the new administrative and economic imperatives. Finally, in his eighties he chose to retire rather than change his definition of appropriate care.

It was before he left the practice of medicine that he and I had a post examination conversation in the late spring of 1991 in which he told me that while I had always had some microscopic traces of blood in my urine, at this visit I had a bit more than usual. He suggested that he call his urologist colleague whom I had already encountered when the first blood appeared some years earlier to determine whether he might want to examine me. Then, almost as quickly as he'd picked the handset up he placed it in its cradle and commented that there really was no point to the phone consultation—that surely the answer to his question would be "yes—and that I should call and set up an appointment.

I did. And so it was that a week later I had an ultra-sound, a procedure with which I was already familiar. As I lay on the examining table, the young, personable technician told me "this will take twenty minutes" and began to move the transducer probe over what I thought was the relevant part of my body. Time went by and it soon was evident that she had extended her search to encompass a wider area. Furthermore, she seemed to be doing some areas a second and third time. She explained that now she was doing the gall bladder, now the kidneys, and so forth. It now was well beyond twenty minutes and though aware that my knowledge of anatomy was quite limited I was increasingly irritated and urged the technician to limit her examination to the "relevant" part of my body. She responded that it was normal procedure to cover a wider area and there was no additional charge for doing so.

Some forty or more minutes after we began she told she had concluded the examination and I rose and quite irritably said, "We live in a weird country." "How so?" she responded. I had had plenty of time to think about it and said, "A weird country is one that claims that it doesn't have the resources to provide health care to all its children and yet has the resources and the equipment and the time to examine all the organs, even ones that have nothing to do with a microscopic bit of blood in urine." I left and was so proud of the way I had "told the health care system off" about its excesses and misallocation of resources that I repeated the story with some pride to relatives who were joining us for dinner that evening. I, the economist, had planted the flag for responsible cost-containment!

Events moved rapidly after the ultrasound. The next day my urologist told me I'd need a cat (CT) scan to determine whether I had a cyst or something more on the wall of my right kidney. Boston's ample supply of health care resources enabled the scan to be done within two days and it was then that the radiologist informed me that it wasn't a cyst and that it would be necessary to operate and remove the kidney. I realized that I had behaved abominably toward the technician. Surely she had seen something troubling and, therefore, had been very careful and deliberate in her wide-ranging examination. Enjoined not to share what she saw with the patient and explain why the examination was especially thorough and lengthy, she had had to put up with my declamations about the wasteful allocation of resources and not grin, but bear it. I suppose I was not the first boor she had encountered, but I wasn't really a boor, just your average cost-conscious and socially responsible, but not very knowledgeable, health care economist.

Surgery took place two weeks later and could have been scheduled even sooner, but for some delays having nothing to do with availability of resources. Things went smoothly. The kidney was removed, the tumor was stage 1 and fully encapsulated. On the third day I turned to the urologist and asked "what will be different from now on." In a book on kidney cancer that I had skimmed in the time that I was waiting for the operation, I had read that some physicians believed that a low protein diet was called for if an individual had only one kidney. I wanted to know whether that was really so and what changes in life style I would face. My urologist responded, "Nothing will be different. Your diet doesn't have to change. But there is one thing: I will want you to have an ultrasound once a year."

I heard myself thinking "Why only once a year? Surely something untoward can happen soon after an ultrasound and we wouldn't know about it for almost a year. Why not every six months and perhaps even oftener?" I didn't dare give voice to my questions and risk my credentials as an economist concerned about cost-containment and the allocation of scarce resources in the most appropriate fashion. But I know I thought that in my case once a year was not often enough, that semi-annually or even quarterly made much more sense. I worked in the Harvard medical area and was surrounded by hospitals; I could come in every day! After all, the perspective of the patient not of the economist—and certainly not of the green-shaded accountant—should guide decisions. I didn't say it, but I did think that perhaps my urologist was worrying a bit too much about health care expenditures and a bit too little about this patient. There was nothing invasive about an ultrasound; the only damage it might do would be to my pocketbook. Indeed, even that was an exaggeration: my pocketbook was not really at risk. I was covered by Medicare and my employer contributed to a Medicare supplement. Why not go for it? The data might say that the chances of finding something were one in a thousand, perhaps as small as one in ten thousand, but the probability was irrelevant: one is greater than zero and someone would be that one. Perhaps it would be I. Why not? In the brief span of two or three weeks I had abandoned the societal viewpoint and adopted that of the individual patient. I had lost a kidney and gained a new perspective.

Of course, I felt I understood the patient's perspective well before I became a patient. As I have already written, I had given the matter much thought, almost from the very first days that I came to Harvard Medical School. I was well aware that my courses, important as they were, would be dwarfed by the attitudes and perspectives of the total curriculum. As a prospective patient—which every one of us is—I didn't really mind the school's emphasis. Nevertheless, the real patient brought a certain emotion to the problem that the imaginary patient did not possess. Yet, even then and still today, I was not and am not ready to dismiss the societal concern. And thus we see the potential conflict. It is both easy and accurate to say that if a medical intervention does nothing for ninety-nine patients while extending life by five years for one, on average life is extended by less than three weeks. Yet it is also accurate for the individual who believes that he or she will be the "survivor"—and that may be the way every one of the one hundred patients feels—to say "Not a single one of the hundred patients will live for five additional weeks. That's a calculated average and may have little to do with me. There is no 'average patient.' Most likely I'll be one of the many who derive no benefit, but perhaps I'll be the one who lives five more years." Nor is it inaccurate to say that many physicians feel the way their patient does and that, as patients, we may want them to feel that way. The fact that society's average perspective and the patient's individual perspective are both in play is the problem.

Consider the following. A university accepts 10 percent of its 400 applicants and rejects 90 percent. Over the typical four year college experience, those accepted will spend 120 weeks (thirty weeks per year for four years) in residence. Those rejected, of course, will spend zero. The forty applicants who become students will spend a total of 4,800 weeks while the remaining 360 rejected applicants will spend zero time at the university. Thus, the so called "average applicant" can look forward to spending a mere twelve weeks, less than one semester, at the college (4,800 weeks divided by 400 applicants). Looked at that way—that is, in the same way that we calculate how long the "average" patient survives—it is hardly worth applying. The social costs are much too high. But, of course, that is not the way applicants look at the problem. She or he considers the private costs and imagines they will be accepted. They know they won't get twelve weeks of time at that college: they'll not be there at all or they will spend a full four years. Indeed, I rather suspect that is the way even the statisticians who discuss survival rates and who calculate that the procedure will extend life by less than three weeks thinks about the admission process when their daughters or sons apply to college.

That the perspectives of the economist policy adviser (who, presumably, has the societal approach) and of the patient (or other target population) are different should come as no surprise. Nor should we be surprised that physicians who face constraints or protocols set by insurers often behave as surrogates for those who set policy. Of course there are inevitable tensions. Both the economist's concern about a resource allocation that maximizes all benefits or some subset of health benefits and the patient's concern with his or her benefits, though what benefits are really available is heavily influenced by the individual's income and quality of insurance coverage, are valid. The tension and problem arise, at least in part, because sometimes the patient's and at other times the economist's perspective wins out and there seems to be little rhyme or reason—except income and ability to pay—to explain who is victorious. Policy makers who try and erect systems that will limit care only to that which is "necessary" should be aware that there will be resistance from affected parties. Some individuals will feel they are being denied services that are of value and that they don't simply desire, but need. Furthermore, if those services are available on the open market to those who can and will pay for them on their own, low-income individuals will not readily accept the fact that they are denied the care because they can't afford to buy it on their own.

Some, perhaps many, patients believe that an additional test, visit, or intervention may prove beneficial and, even if skeptical about the benefits of another visit or another test, the physician does not want to play the role of "gatekeeper," the one to say "no." Furthermore, the physician may feel the need to practice "defensive medicine" have a monetary stake in ordering one more test—especially, of course, if he or she owns the diagnostic equipment—and may reap a monetary reward from one more visit. As a consequence, insurers believe that their task is to monitor utilization and to control costs, if necessary, by denying claims even if the patient and physician believe the additional medical care would or might be helpful. Of course, there is a certain symmetry and consequent tension for just as the physician may increase income by ordering one more test, so the insurance company may increase its profits by saying "No."

It is not surprising that the issues of health expenditures and payment and reimbursement mechanisms that might help control expenditures are the preoccupation of many policy analysts. I was fortunate that my insurer was loath to interfere with my physician's clinical judgment and that my physician practiced by older rules and ordered additional tests instead of waiting six months to see how things went. I became doubly aware of my good fortune when some time after the surgery, my urologist reported that in spite of the removal of the kidney my urine still contained traces of blood. We had found the kidney cancer by accident

That different persons with different backgrounds and different responsibilities are likely to have different perspectives is not a startling observation. What was unusual in this case is that I embodied both perspectives at virtually the same time. That, in fact, is the very problem that many physicians face. Society wants the physician to intervene only when appropriate (a somewhat elusive standard), and conserve resources. It exerts pressure to that end.

An increasing number of medical students are exposed to that way of thinking about problems. Yet at the same time, patients expect the physician to be their advocate and "work" on their behalf. With multiple allegiances, today's physician is being asked to at one and the same time stand at the patient's bed side and while doing so represent society, a recipe that may increase the number of schizophrenic physicians.

It is important that we understand the attitudes the various participants in the medical care drama—the patient, physician, hospital director, epidemiologist, statistician, insurance company executive, employer, government budget analyst, regulator, policy adviser, and others—bring to the issue of resource use. One's attitudes may differ depending on the role that each of us is playing. And it becomes exceedingly complex when, as is often the case, we play multiple roles. What may appear to be a frivolous use of resources to one may seem too constraining to others—or as with me, to the same individual at different times. Whatever the answer to the allocation issue and to the tensions thus generated, I believe one thing is quite certain: in this arena (as in other arenas) differences in perspective and the inevitable tensions such differences generate are not likely to be resolved unless we all do a better job of listening to others, understanding their points of view, and incorporating the various judgments in the development of public policy.

Comments that Increase Our Understanding

Sometimes comments that appear irrelevant to policy considerations may reveal an individual's value orientation and thus enrich the adviser's understanding and potential effectiveness. Just such an incident occurred in March of 1978 at a meeting Senator Edward Kennedy held on national health insurance at his home in McLain, Virginia. Kennedy had a long and rich history of support of universal health care. In 1970 he had sponsored the Kennedy-Griffiths bill which, in today's terminology would have been classified as a "single-payer" or "Medicare for All" social-insurance measure. In 1974 he and Representative Wilbur Mills had developed the Kennedy-Mills compromise legislation as an alternative to President Nixon's Family Health Insurance Program. When President

Carter took office and indicated his potential support for a universal program while setting various constraints on program characteristics (for example, preserving an underwriting role for the private commercial insurance industry) Kennedy responded by asking his staff and a few outside advisers/consultants—I was among the latter—to develop a new piece of legislation that would embody the characteristics the president had deemed essential while addressing those matters the senator deemed vital, especially issues of progressivity and of triggers and timing. That was the genesis of the Senator's "Health Care for All Americans Act."

I was to make a presentation of this new initiative at a dinner for a number of labor leaders at the senator's home. Some of us who had worked closely with the senator were asked to come early and we gathered in front of the fireplace for some conversation. After a bit, Doug Fraser, the president of the United Automobile Workers (UAW) whom I had come to know when he was chairman of the Committee for National Health Insurance and I was the chairman of its Technical Committee, turned to me and said that he, of course, had read about the Nor'easter that dumped over twenty-seven inches of snow on the greater Boston area on February 6-7, 1978 and that paralyzed the city. I was the first Bostonian Frazier had met since the blizzard and he wondered what it really had been like. I responded that, perhaps surprisingly, I found it a rather pleasant experience. As it happened, because of an impending trip I had not brought any work home from the office. Since it was before the home computer days, the sense of isolation from possible work was quite real and quite different from that which would prevail today. Except for emergency vehicles, automobile travel was banned. As a consequence, I did a lot of reading, catching up on things around the house, taking care of correspondence, and so forth. I continued with a description of taking late-afternoon walks with my wife through the clean air and clean snow and, forgetting that I was talking to the head of the UAW, commented on how pleasant it was not to have any cars or automobile pollution around: everything was cleaner, quieter, and safer. Then, after the walk, my wife and I sat in front of the fire in the fireplace and had a scotch. In short, the week of enforced idleness, long walks and short scotches and an occasional short walk and long scotch, all without the usual guilt, added up to a rather pleasant experience.

Perhaps it was the almost idyllic way I described the event, perhaps it was because he sensed that others were enjoying my experience vicariously, almost wishing they had a week of enforced "vacation," long walks, and fireplace drinks, Senator Kennedy turned to—perhaps, the more appropriate word is "on"—me and in a tone I had not previously heard in our relationship, with restrained anger in his voice and demeanor said something like: "Pleasant, you say. You describe it as pleasant, relaxing, almost like fun. Let me tell you that I had the experience of flying in a helicopter over the coastline in order to survey the damage caused by the high tides and the Nor'easter winds that pushed the water onto the coast line and over both natural and man-made barriers. High on the cliffs, far above water's edge, are the large homes and mansions, the kinds of places in which—did he say "rich folks" or "folks like the Kennedys"—live. Perhaps those people also had what you call a pleasant experience. But below, at water's edge, where the 'ordinary' people live, the waters came in at high tide pushed by winds with blowing snow, that's where homes were washed away. At water's edge people lost their homes and even when those survived lost their belongings." As I remember he ended with a sharp "So don't ever describe it as a pleasant week."

I cannot vouch that those were Senator Kennedy's exact words, but I am certain those were the ideas he conveyed. I am equally certain that he did not present his description of events as if he were reading from a column of data that I had somehow overlooked or in some analytic manner devoid of emotion and involvement. Perhaps it was not even that he was angry at what I said, but at what I didn't say. I had not spoken of the pain, the suffering, the homes destroyed and lives altered. I had not spoken about the "ordinary" people. I had not shown awareness or empathy and had presented a distorted picture of the event. He, who was far more privileged than I, felt he needed to remind me that events, policies, and perhaps especially disasters, have vastly different implications for people in different socio-economic circumstances. He spoke instinctively and with passion. I could not help being reminded of

Robert F. Kennedy's reactions during his examination of hunger and poverty in Mississippi. Both brothers showed us they cared and neither thought there was some virtue in hiding their emotions, in appearing to be "tough." Those of us around the fireplace who heard Ted Kennedy speak about the distributional impact of a weather event knew he was authentic. I am not certain I had ever encountered a similar situation. Talk to him about a blizzard and he saw it through a distributional prism: who escaped and who was hurt and what determined into which group folks fell. I was not with Ted Kennedy in the days after Katrina. Yet I feel I know what he was thinking and the questions he was asking of his staff.

The reader may ask "So what? What's the point"? Is this merely an interesting tale about a famous senator who even then, over thirty years ago, was an important force in American political affairs? Even if that were all, it might be worth retelling, but I believe there is much more. I may have thought of it that night; I know that I have thought of it many times since. I believe that my colleagues who are political scientists may have no more important and difficult task than to devise mechanisms and situations that enable us, the general public, the voters, to assess what an incumbent legislator or executive and/or a candidate feels in his or her gut. We want and need to know where people stand and are aware that today's policy positions may not be tomorrow's. We know that new and unanticipated issues may arise and that under new conditions and with new knowledge elected officials may need to change their priorities. Because we cannot predict what unanticipated events may occur, we must guess how those who need to make decisions will react.

Thus, we are aware that we must listen carefully, watch for nuances, and guess. We are seldom fortunate enough to be up close and be certain that we can sense "authenticity." We do know that authenticity cannot be programmed and we seek to understand what candidates really feel, to what they react and how they do so. In a system in which the party has come to mean less and the individual has become more independent, it becomes increasingly necessary to know the individual in a way that makes it possible to assess where he or she is likely to stand on issues that have not yet surfaced. Perhaps the "little things," for example, how individuals think about blizzards and their impacts, would tell us how they might think about Katrina. Is it too much of a stretch to imagine that how one thinks about the distributional impact of a blizzard might help us predict how one might think about expanding Head Start or about national health insurance? Retelling the stories reminds me of the importance of trying to discern the prism through which leaders filter events and how those events affect them. It reminds us of the importance of "values."

It almost goes without saying there is a second reason to retell the story of the blizzard. It is useful—and, as with me that evening, sometimes necessary—to be reminded that any assessment of the impact of events or of policy must take account of the wide diversity of those affected. Not all of us are taking long walks in the clean snow and sitting in front of the fire. We are not all living high on the cliffs. Most of us are "little" people even though most of those who study and plan public policy initiatives, who legislate and enact appropriations, who fly to inspect the effects of blizzards, hurricanes, floods, and fires have above average incomes, above average education, above average entrée into the offices of those with power. We who know how the system works and who are able to work the system need to remember that events and policies have very different implications for "others," for people who fall in very different socio-economic groupings. I had worked with Senator Kennedy for almost a decade and knew where he stood on any number of issues. Even so, I learned something important that evening: why he stood where he did. It was instructive to hear and understand the instinctive reflex reaction.

But the remainder of the evening presented yet another lesson: one dare not value a proposed course of action simply because one agrees with its goals and objectives. It is easy—and wrong—to support a legislative initiative simply because proponents claim it would help make life a little less unfair. Programs have to be designed in ways that work. That became the subject of the conversation when we gathered for dinner and for the presentation of the structure of the proposed Health Care for All Americans Act, an admittedly complex piece of legislation designed to be a compromise between what we knew was the senator's position and what we believed was the president's. It had to satisfy two masters.

There are at least two problems with complexity: the first is whether the complex proposal can be understood, a very real problem as President Clinton learned fifteen year later from the Harry and Louise attack on his Health Security Act; the second is whether it can work. The latter question has to deal with the fact that every step in a complex arrangement creates one more situation in which "error" can be introduced. If there are enough steps—for example: some approaches to universal coverage may involve registration of the beneficiary and of the employer, verification of income, payment of premium, recording of medical condition as well as changes in demographic attributes such as income and employment—the total error rate at the end of the required steps can be quite considerable, even if the error rate for each individual step is quite low.

I worked hard to simplify the presentation of a complicated piece of legislation. Nevertheless, I could not hide the fact that it was complicated: less so, perhaps, than a Rube Goldberg creation, but complicated nonetheless. Perhaps sensing that some of the people around the table needed reassurance that it all made sense, perhaps wanting me to say something to indicate that we were aware of the complexity and felt that we had dealt with it, whatever the reason, when I completed my remarks the senator turned and asked "But will it work?" He had held numerous and detailed discussion about the bill and its many characteristics, knew the legislation quite well and had "signed off" on it, but I believe he wanted everyone to understand that the question was not whether the goal was worthy, but whether the mechanism would get us to our objective. Stating a worthy objective may make one feel good, but reaching the objective is what effective policy is about. The senator was reminding us that the Health Care for All Americans Act was not a proposal we should support simply because it and we were on the side of the righteous. We had to believe it would work. My answer was to help make clear that even though complicated, it could be implemented successfully.

I believe that the two tales that took place in the Kennedy home are paired appropriately and by more than the fact that they occurred in virtually the same location within the space of a very few hours. To me, the first stresses the importance of remembering and caring about the vast number of people, our neighbors, who live on the edge. It also stresses the value of understanding the lens through which our representatives see issues. It is not irrelevant in understanding Senator Kennedy that he saw things through the lens of distributional equity. Almost instinctively the question he asked in processing information is "Is it fair and can I make it fairer?" But the story about the explanation of the Health Care for All Americans Act is also of value in emphasizing that wanting to "do good" is not enough. It is not enough to want to make the world a better place; it is not enough to suggest programs that one believes might do so. Designing the "best" health financing program, education or housing program is easy if we remove all real world constraints. But programs that one advocates as solutions to real world problems need to be subjected to rigorous analysis. The policy adviser must ask, "but will it work?" That question is no less important than the question "is it fair?" It was an accident that both stories happened on the same evening. It is no accident that in telling them I see a logical as well as a temporal connection.

I recall another incident, one that may have been equally revealing. Early in President Nixon's administration two colleagues and I, all health economists, were invited to meet with various officials representing the Council of Economic Advisers, the Bureau of the Budget, the Department of Health, Education, and Welfare, and White House staff to conduct an all day seminar on medical economics. It was a long and tiring day. The discussion was wide ranging and, among other things, examined the philosophical underpinnings of Medicare and Medicaid. We discussed the differences between and effectiveness of "universal" programs (as in Medicare and Social Security) and "targeted" programs (as in Medicaid and welfare) and the contrasting views of the role of government in explaining and assessing those differences. The three of us argued in favor of the Medicare approach, in part, because it strengthened "social cohesion." Conversely, most if not all the various administration representatives felt that the Medicare program should have been limited to the poor elderly. Perhaps, however, just as in March of 1978 I learned about the attitudes and values of Senator Kennedy by his reaction to comments I made about weather, so I learned about a very different thought pattern from one of the White House participants at the meeting.

As our dinner in the White House Mess was ending—I refer to a dining room not a situation—the person who had invited me to join in the seminar rose to escort me to a White House car that would get me to the airport in time for the last Boston flight of the day. My "escort" intervened when I reached for the door-handle on the front passenger's side, telling me that I should sit in the back. I responded that I had been in White House cars before—I saw no need to add "infrequently"—and that now, as then, I preferred to sit up front and talk to the driver. I again reached for the handle and felt a hand clamp down on mine. Drawing a sharp contrast with where I sat those other times, my escort coldly and very deliberately said, "In this administration you'll sit in the back." I regret I did not fully appreciate what a revealing commentary this was on his (and some might argue, the administration's) value system and how his words encompassed his view on the perquisites of power. The simple words about where to ride told me more than I recognized at the time. I am certain that they had colored the dialogue that we had engaged in earlier in the day and I wish I had known that at the time. Understanding the value orientations of the various participants would have enabled a richer discussion. In retrospect it was clear that my escort's views and mine about medical economics were as much about values as about analyses. Regrettably, those issues were not explored or joined.

Policy advisers must be aware of the values they hold as well as those held by those with whom they intersect. Without that knowledge many conversations will fail to get to the heart of the problem and provide little illumination of the basis for agreements and disagreements. Policy advisers who recognize, as good policy advisers must, that part of their task is to anticipate requests and not simply react to issues raised by the person for and with whom they work, must know their principals well enough to know what issues they should think about and the framework, the lens, through which to view the issues they confront. Sometimes, simple words:

"So don't ever describe it as a pleasant week," "But will it work," "In this administration you'll sit in the back" reveal important truths. We must listen for them.

5

Four Lessons

The Known Drives Out the Abstract

Just as defining the encompassing reach of a policy objective is of vital importance, so it is also critical to exercise care in defining the population that would be directly and indirectly affected by the proposal in question and to ask whether one has selected the appropriate target. Does the policy fall within the jurisdiction of the decision maker? Is the affected population one for which the decision maker is responsible? How does one define one's constituency? We are quite familiar with variants of this problem which arise at the different levels of government because many of our representatives are elected by geographic constituencies each of which is smaller than the area for which the totality of representatives is responsible. The full House of Representatives is responsible to the nation even as each representative is elected within a congressional district. Senators are selected by the electorate within a state, but they serve in a body that legislates on behalf of the nation. Some city councilors may run "at large," but others are elected by wards. Is the allegiance of the latter to the city? Most assuredly. Is their allegiance to their ward? Of course. How are these sometimes conflicting responsibilities to be met? Even the president and vice president are not elected by a popular vote, but by a process that takes geography into account. In all cases, the policy adviser must know whom his principal feels he or she is representing.

The issue of whom a policy affects and whom the decision maker represents is not one unique to government. The private sector is not immune from the same phenomenon and the policy maker must be sensitive to the issues raised. This is no trivial matter. I served on the board of trustees of a hospital affiliated with the Harvard Medical School. The board met every few months and it was rewarding to see the commitment by successful and busy lay individuals to an "extra-curricular" activity that yielded no personal financial benefit—perhaps, however, the nurses were more solicitous when a trustee was hospital-ized—but which provided an opportunity to strengthen a community enterprise. At such meetings we heard a report from the general direc-tor, from the person in charge of finance, and various others with important, including clinical, responsibilities.

Over the years—and not unrelated to the state of the American medical enterprise—the proportion of time devoted to financial matters increased and the proportion of time devoted to reports that dealt with matters of quality, with new procedures, or with issues of what might be termed "community affairs"—including potential affiliation with community health centers—decreased. In general, the meetings were interesting and, on occasion, provoca-tive. Thus, for example, we had a somewhat heated and certainly lengthy discussion on whether to have a flat and high charge or an income related scale of charges for non-insured in-vitro-fertilization procedures. Nevertheless, everyone recognized that most important decisions were made by a much smaller executive committee and that, most often, our role was to ratify those decisions.

On one occasion we were told that we would enter into execu-tive session because the matter that would be discussed was highly charged and needed to be treated as confidential. We were informed that a physician with privileges in our institution had been with two close physician friends who practiced in the same specialty as he, but who were associated with another hospital. "Our" physician suggested that his friends should seek privileges at our institution: "We're a nice bunch of guys and you know many of us. We'd enjoy welcoming you and you'd enjoy being associated with us." The invitation was issued with a clear implication that there would not be any problem if the individuals applied. The motivation was friendship rather than the desire to add to staff and thereby perhaps generate more patients and fill more beds.

The physicians did apply and when the applications were received the hospital exercised due diligence and examined the relevant credentials and performance. Unfortunately, the responsible medical committee concluded that in each case the individual's performance was sorely lacking, that neither one performed at a standard that would reflect favorably upon the hospital, and that we would be taking a considerable risk if we accepted their applications. While not revealing the name of the individuals in question, we were told that since they were respected and well-known members of the general community, we might hear about the matter and it would be good for us to have this bit of background.

In summary: we knew that physicians associated with another hospital were performing at a standard that our institution felt was unacceptable, indeed, as described, dangerous to those patients whom they treated. Yet, though we knew the name of the hospital where they practiced, we did not know the names of the physicians. One trustee raised her hand and asked for the physicians' names: "If these men are a danger to their patients, I want to make certain that I don't seek care from them." The request was turned down because divulging names might have legal implications and the trustee's concerns could be met another way: "Don't worry. The way to make certain you aren't treated by either one of them is to avoid the hospital in which they practice and that is easily done by continuing to get your in-hospital care from this institution." That led to a follow-up inquiry: whether we were going to share our findings with the other institution within whose walls the physicians practiced. After all, what of our friends and relatives who might seek care, what of all the other patients who were at risk? Did we not owe them some responsibility? Was our concern to be limited to us and to "our" patients or were we concerned about and even responsible to the larger community? The answer was that we would not share any information that could lead to a suit and legal costs. Apparently the dictum "do no harm" applied to what happened within our hospital's walls, but not outside and not to unknown patients. We defined our mission to promote better health in quite narrow terms.

This attitude, regrettably, is not uncommon. Policy makers often operate in their own self-interest. They may believe that if everyone has the same information and the same capacity to act upon it, the sum of all self-interest motivated actions will advance the entire society. Those assumptions, however, are unrealistic. In the real world those who pursue their own self-interest instead of exhibiting concern for other members of the larger community, may place their neighbors at risk. If "our" hospital—a not-for-profit community enterprise—worries only about what happens inside its walls, who guards health care for the community?

I once spoke to a meeting of a state medical society on the role of the physician and of government and the perceived conflict between them. During the question and answer part of the program it became clear that the perspective of most of the two hundred or so physicians in the room was that government was intrusive and irresponsible, that its regulations were adding to the physician's burdens, and that life would be simpler and better both for patients and physicians if government were less active in the health care sector. No one acknowledged that through Medicare and Medicaid government had relieved the physician from the onus of having to ration care and therapeutic interventions on the basis of the patient's ability to pay. No one acknowledged that many of the constraints they complained about were placed on physicians by insurance companies and reflected the role that private employers played in purchasing employee health insurance. Put simply: government was "the enemy."

I found myself asking how many in the audience knew a physician in whom they had so little confidence that—shades of the clichéd idiom of the South—they wouldn't want their sister to have him as an MD. Most of the assembled raised their hands. I then asked whether, acting through their medical society, they were prepared to do something about those incompetent and dangerous practitioners. I was about to suggest that if they wouldn't act, then they had little grounds for objecting to government action to protect the greater community. But before I could get all the words out, the president of the society left his chair, rushed to the microphone, and intervened: "Before you agree that the medical society ought to act, consider whether you are willing to have your dues raised by a significant amount. If you would have us act, be prepared to finance the legal action in which we will surely become involved. How many of you are willing to have your dues go up?" If the vote on "bad" physicians was almost unanimous, the vote against the willingness to face a dues increase was equally unanimous. Apparently, the price to be paid to achieve transparency was too high.

In each of the two cases I recount the issue was what to do about protecting prospective patients from physicians whose standards of performance were such that they could be considered as dangers to the community. In neither case was anyone prepared to take the kind of action that would attempt to protect the community. In both cases the reason given for rejecting that approach was the threat of legal entanglements. That threat may well have been real: taking the kind of action that can disbar a member of a profession and thus the right to earn a livelihood at one's profession is no trivial matter. One should expect a "push back." Nevertheless, that may not be the true explanatory variable. Legal risks and consequences can be dealt with, but I believe that something else much more basic was at play, something that policy advisers must be aware of and on guard against.

It relates to the form that empathy may take, to the issue of responsibility, and to the ability to balance the interests of the individual or organization we know and with which we are familiar—our "buddies" –against those of individuals who are anonymous and unknown to us. Of course, we are prepared to act to protect ourselves and family members from some physicians—we know those potential patients. We will also act to protect the organizations we belong to—in a sense they are "us." These stand in sharp contrast to the much larger body of patients who, faceless and nameless, are more readily ignored. This ability to ignore those who are "mere" or abstract—faceless and nameless—statistics and, in doing so, to forget one's mission and in a policy sense, serve the wrong target population, was brought home in the behavior of a promotions committee on which I served.

The case involved a medical student who hadn't performed well in his clinical encounters, had been given a "second chance," and was still doing poorly. It was clear that his various instructors had warned him and had discussed their deep misgivings about his abilities and his future as a practicing physician. It also was clear that none of the members of the promotions committee doubted the judgment of the physicians who had evaluated him. Nevertheless they did not want to take the action that I, a non-physician, believed was called for. They sought to avoid issuing the harsh invitation to leave, to find some basis for giving the student yet one more chance.

Perhaps, a small part of the phenomenon was related to the "doctrine of the infallibility of the admissions committee." Surely, it hadn't committed an error when the young man was admitted to Harvard. Obviously, he must have possessed the requisite abilities. It, therefore, followed that something must have gone wrong after he came and the school's task was to discern what that was and then to intervene and—as physicians so often do with patients—save him. The "don't give up" syndrome was at work. One could not help but admire the commitment. Neither could one ignore the possibility that the student would continue to underperform and yet slip through the system and be permitted to graduate and enter medical practice.

I had encountered the doctrine of infallibility some time earlier. I once told a Harvard associate dean that there was a certain irony in the fact that here I was at Harvard as a full professor in a university that had not admitted me when I applied for undergraduate admission. The associate dean quickly commented that obviously Harvard had made a mistake, a conclusion with which I concurred telling him I was sure that, if admitted, I would have graduated. But I was told I misunderstood: the mistake he referred to was in awarding me the professorship. Because of the "doctrine of the infallibility of the admissions committee," the error that occurred was made when I was invited to join the faculty.

Yet, I believe that the real explanation for the behavior of the promotions committee in wanting to give the young man as many chances as it would take for him to "pass," was the contrast between the abstraction "the patients he will encounter" and the real-life student whom many of the committee members knew—and if they didn't know him personally, they knew him as one of "us." The prospective patients did not have names; our student did. When the issue about the committee's responsibility to the abstract concept called "society" and to the anonymous patients the young man would see if he were granted his degree was raised, it did remind the committee of the need to consider all the "populations" at risk. But the issue had to be raised; it did not come naturally.

Certainly, the threat of legal action played a role in the behavior of the hospital and of the medical society. Perhaps it even influenced the promotions committee. But I believe that part of the dynamic is the result of "specificity" being more significant in guiding policy than the amorphous and in some sense unknown. The power of the news article that focuses on the anecdote, on the individual, and on the case is far more compelling that the academic journal article that, at best, discusses the group and at worst eschews the discussion and presents tables of data. The speaker who begins with the human interest story of the individual who has been evicted, has lost her insurance, or is trying to deal with the complex choices available under Medicare Part D stands a chance of capturing the audience's attention. The speaker who begins with national statistics about faceless people is operating under a significant, even if self-imposed, handicap. He or she has to rely on the audience to make the leap from the somewhat "dry" data to flesh and blood human beings.

The policy adviser must consider whom his policy will affect and in what manner. Even as he or she recognizes the various constituencies and the fact that some are more closely related than others to the decision maker, account must be taken of those others who are less well known, less able to make their voices heard, and, as a consequence, less well represented. The task of the policy adviser is to make certain that they receive the attention they merit and that they are not ignored simply because they are anonymous.

Not Everyone Thinks Like an Economist

Policy analysts and advisers are not fools. However limited their perspective may be when they first embark on their activity, they will soon learn that colleagues with different skills, backgrounds, and experiences may, and often do, provide valuable insights. If that escapes their attention they likely will discover that they must seek other employment. Nevertheless, there will be occasions—for example, a time constrained emergency or the need for confidentiality—when they must rely on their own judgment and fund of knowledge. When that occurs they may choose to call upon the same methodology that many of us rely on when thinking about areas about which we may not be sufficiently knowledgeable and, therefore, are somewhat uncomfortable. That methodology is especially appealing when trying to guess at behavioral responses to a set of changing circumstances. I refer to introspection -- a powerful, but at the same time, a dangerous analytic tool. Thus, if I do not know how others might feel, let me guess by examining how I might feel.

In trying to understand how people might react to different incentives, it seems quite plausible for an adviser to begin an inquiry by looking inward and considering how he or she might react or behave under similar circumstances and assuming that the way he or she would react is the way others would as well. Doing that may be quite appealing and may seem close to that which I suggested earlier: imagine you are the "other." Yet, it is worlds apart. Suggesting one should try to imagine he or she is the "other" is clearly not the same as assuming that others are like you. One may gain some—perhaps, considerable—insight by imagining what it is like to be a stevedore, an African-American, or an uninsured individual. But the converse does not hold: by imagining how you might behave under certain conditions one will gain little insight into the behavior of stevedores, African-Americans, or the uninsured. There is little reason to presume that their behavior would be similar to what you imagine—but in fact are not even certain—your own would be. Put simply, one cannot assume one's own behavior or reaction to events is "typical." The same incentives may play upon each of us in different ways. Attitudes will vary with gender, age, income, wealth, national origin, ethnic and religious identification. Attitudes are shaped by cultural backgrounds and other socio-economic and demographic characteristics and attitudes are likely to influence behavior.

Nevertheless, individuals are often tempted to assume that others would react as they would in similar situations. That may be especially the case when they view their behavior as appropriate and consistent with a general theoretic structure. Thus, economists who react to a set of incentives in what they consider to be a rational economic manner are likely to assume that not only other economists but other "sensible" folk would react and behave the same way. The former have taken the same courses, learned the same theory, and are likely to think as economists think. Economists are tempted to, and do, assume that the latter, the non-economists, though unaware that they are doing so, behave in ways that follow certain more or less predictable (and appropriate) patterns of economic response. Indeed, if that were not the case, if there were no *homo economicus,* much of economic analysis would be fallacious. Economists have a stake in assuming that there is an "economic man," Yet one may be led astray in deferring too much to that one construct. We are bundles of many things: we are economic, altruistic, friendly, loving, grasping, daring, spiteful, boisterous, frivolous, and many more.

Many years ago I attended a conference on health care in which one session was devoted to a discussion of the potential increase in demand for health care as a result of expansion of insurance benefits, decreases in cost-sharing, and an increase in the number of "covered" individuals. There was agreement that more and broader insurance would increase access to and utilization of medical care even including some that was "unnecessary." Indeed, some conferees seemed to believe that if the monetary cost of an additional physician visit were lowered to zero the demand for visits would explode, that at a zero price the demand would be infinite.

How much demand for care would expand—the size of the explosion—was an empirical question, but absent the data, individuals could and did disagree, a phenomenon that sometimes occurs even in the presence of data. Some believed that the increase in demand might be quite modest. Colleagues who had worked in inner-city hospital outpatient departments had often commented on the impediments to the continuity of care and to effective disease prevention and health promotion activities even when the monetary cost of a follow-up visit was zero. They spoke about the need to mount outreach services and special efforts to get patients to use their prescribed medications and to return for treatment and follow up. It was not clear whether the problem with return visits was the loss of time and wages, the cost of medications or of transportation, or that the patients were afraid that the physician would confirm their worst fears: the irrational, but not uncommon view that one isn't sick till the doctor says so. Those out-patient physicians knew that their patients did not consider visiting a doctor as one of the more enjoyable ways to spend one's time or money. Even so, there was general agreement that though we might not know the size of the increase, we certainly could assume there would be some growth in utilization. Some of it might be unnecessary, but much of it would be welcome. That, after all, is one of the purposes of expanding the insurance pool.

More physician visits and more hospital stays would most probably lead to an in increase in health expenditures: physicians and hospitals do expect to be paid. In turn, and depending on the way care was financed, higher expenditures would likely lead to higher insurance premiums. These premiums would not reflect the behavior of any one individual, but the consequences of the totality of behaviors. The argument that was advanced was that as a consequence of the increase in monthly premium payments, some—perhaps many—individuals would use more medical services: after all, since they were paying higher premiums they would feel justified in wanting and utilizing more care, in "getting their money's worth." Additionally, some individuals would increase their utilization simply because they believed their neighbors would do so and would not want to be "taken advantage of."

One of the most distinguished economists present tried to get others to understand this phenomenon by describing a situation many of us had experienced and that he believed was analogous. We were asked to think how we would behave if a group of us went to a fine restaurant for dinner and agreed with the waiter's suggestion that we put the bill on a single check that represented the sum of all our orders. Our colleague argued that, aware that the check would be divided equally—the equivalent of the monthly premium—each of us would have an incentive to order the expensive lobster. We might do so in order to take advantage of the opportunity to have someone else share in the cost of an item we liked, but wouldn't normally order because of the expense. Alternatively, we might do so because each of us anticipated that the others would order the lobster and, unless we also did so, when the bill was divided equally we'd find that we were "subsidizing" the others—paying for their lobsters and not having any ourselves. This anticipated behavior may well have been the reason the waiter encouraged us to put the bill on one check. Perhaps she understood the issue because she was an unemployed economist or economics graduate student making ends meet. Perhaps she or he had learned out of experience or observation that placing everything on one check would induce the behavior described and thus a higher total bill and, as a consequence, a larger tip.

On the face of it, the description of our likely behavior made a good deal of sense, and might have appealed to a policy analyst or adviser who was thinking about health care and health insurance. But there were at least two problems. The first related to the weakness of arguing from an analogy that assumes that behavior in the physician's office is the same as or very similar to behavior in a restaurant. Though many do like lobster or other expensive dishes, the comparison of that kind of desirable consumption with a visit to a physician's office is not entirely persuasive.

As already noted, many patients—even including ones who might enjoy lobster—don't like going to the doctor. Furthermore, some information may be missing. What do I learn if I find that in observing restaurant behavior I notice that one or more of the diners did not order a lobster or the "substitute" expensive steak? Perhaps the situation is not explained by an odd response to the presumed incentives, but by the fact that the diners were observant Jews or vegans. Both lobster and steak were off limits. Does the analogy succeed or fail in the face of this information? We do not know.

The second problem deals with the danger of introspection. It also bears examination, for while we are aware that we should be on guard when arguing from analogy, the introspection approach seems sensible and logical. We know how we'd behave and it does not seem unreasonable to assume that others would be of like mind. Yet it, too, can lead us and policy advisers astray. For example, we are aware of instances when we have behaved in a manner opposite than that described. We can easily construct a very different scenario.

Imagine that a party of four who are good friends go to dinner and agree to a single check anticipating that at the conclusion of the meal it will be split equally. The first one to order does not want to take advantage of the friends who will have to pay three-quarters the bill. Though he might well prefer the expensive steak and would be willing to pay for it, he doesn't want to impose the cost on the others. He orders something that is mid-range in price. One of his friends orders next and aware of the price range that has been set by the first order, follows suit. He might have preferred spending an extra ten dollars for the steak, but considers it bad taste to force his friend who has already ordered the seventeen-dollar pasta special to pay the extra amount as his share of the total bill. Ordering independently everyone might have had steak; ordering on one check they all end up with pasta. Total expenditures are less than they would otherwise be; the waiter ends up with a smaller tip.

My colleague reached one conclusion through introspection; I reached a different one. He may find my behavior "irrational" and I may find his insensitive. Of course, eating in a party of four is not the same as sharing insurance costs with thousands of anonymous strangers, but neither is a restaurant meal the same as a physician visit. My colleague may have assumed that most people would behave as he. That assumption has to be tested since few of us are motivated solely by economic considerations. The policy adviser must guard against such theorizing and must check presuppositions against real world data.

This "problem" is not unique to the health field. I discovered that when I was seated next to a colleague on a plane going to Washington. He was on his way to a meeting of a committee that was examining the tax code treatment of philanthropic contributions. During our conversation he asked whether I was aware of the favorable treatment of charitable contributions for those filing an IRS 1040 long form which provided the opportunity to itemize deductions. I replied that I knew that I could deduct charitable contributions and recognized that when I did so, I reduced my federal income tax. Thus, the dollar that I gave to charity did not cost me a dollar. If I were in the 28 percent bracket a $100 gift reduced my taxes by $28 and effectively cost me only $72. To the next question: "Do you give more because of the deduction?" I quickly responded "yes."

His next question went to the issue of possible changes in tax policy: "So if the tax code eliminated the deduction for charitable giving, you would give less wouldn't you?" This, of course, is the argument that not-for-profit charities invoke in making their case against tax code changes that would limit charitable deductions. I did not take more than a moment to respond that I would give more rather than less if the deduction were eliminated. Certain that I had misunderstood, my colleague repeated the question. In turn, I repeated my answer. More than puzzled he asked me to explain how it could be that I increased my charitable gifts because they were deductible and would increase them if the deduction were eliminated. I responded that it seemed obvious to me. I explained that I gave more because of the deduction since the "price" or cost of my gift was reduced by the amount saved in taxes. I was aware that many people, perhaps especially if they are large donors in upper income brackets, would behave that way. I rather suspected, therefore, that if the deduction were eliminated many people—again, perhaps especially large donors—would cut their gifts. That would mean that the various organizations I supported would face budget crises. These organizations tended to be in the human service areas; they could not postpone meeting the current needs of the persons they assisted. If other donors cut back on their gifts as I presumed they would, that meant I would have to give more. In some odd way my answer seemed very logical: I gave more when because of tax implications it cost me less to give and gave more when the needs of not-for-profit agencies increased.

Of course, I do not assert that my response was the norm. Indeed, the rationale I offered—that gifts to human service agencies would drop if the deduction were eliminated—makes clear I felt my behavior was atypical. Neither do I believe that my increase, even if combined with that of others who increased their gift as the charity's deficit rose, would make up for the loss of one large donor's gift.

Nevertheless, as my response made sense to me, I believed it would make sense to more than a few others. An economic model that assumed universal economic rationality and assumed away my and similar behaviors was incomplete and misleading. Those who help make policy must remember that there is more to life than economics; the phrase "economic behavior" is not a synonym for "human behavior." To deny the importance of economics in explaining human behavior is the height of foolishness. So, too, however is the view that economics is sufficient to explain all of our responses to the world that surrounds us and within which we function. The virtues of introspection in alerting analysts to interesting areas for inquiry are evident. Even so, there is a risk that those educated in a particular discipline may make an unwarranted assumption that others think the way they do. Economists, political scientists, and sociologists dare not assume that the general public analyzes economic, political, and social problems in the same manner as they do.

Politics Trumps Rational Economics

As I look back on the subjects that have interested me over the years and on the reasons that I wandered into economics I realize that, though I very much enjoyed the logic and beauty of mathematics, most especially that of geometry and, therefore, of microeconomics, I was never comfortable or satisfied with the view that economics is no more nor less than a series of proofs of theoretic propositions devoid of cultural, historical, or political context. That view, the assumption that there is an "economic man," a *homo economicus,* whose behavior is guided by his responses to a set of economic incentives and constraints, provided the underpinning of my undergraduate and graduate economic education. Though recent work by behavioral economists increase the applicability of economics to "real" world issues and questions by asking how people behave rather than assuming that question away, the notion of the economic rational actor remains a central analytic tool and guiding principle.

Of course, one dare not reject economic analysis simply because it abstracts from the real world. All of us engage in abstraction because we need and have theoretical structures that help in classifying some facts as important and influential and others as irrelevant. We do not fault the historian who tells us about the weather on July 1-3, 1863 at Gettysburg and who ignores conditions in Charleston and Cleveland. The former may be relevant to the outcome of the battle; no theoretic structure suggests the latter are. The issue before the economist and policy adviser is not whether to exclude, but what to exclude. French, British, Swedish, and U.S. economists may be very much alike in their understanding of economic principles and analytic techniques, but their societies have applied those principles quite differently and each has constructed its own set of socio-economic arrangements. Clearly, culture, history, politics, and the weights to be accorded different values and choices, do make a difference. Though the discipline is called "economics," once we enter the world of application and of economic policy we have entered the world of political economy. That world, as I have stated earlier, is a world that calls upon our knowledge and understanding of other disciplines, such as sociology, psychology, and political science, as well as the institutions in the applied field itself.

Three incidents can serve to illustrate the difference between the economist's pure logic and the realities of the political world in which the application of that logic is embedded. All three relate to policy decisions made in the private sector. The first two involve the labor movement; the third involve corporate leadership and corporate behavior. When each incident occurred I applied my economic reasoning and could not help but conclude that I must be missing something. After all, the various decision makers were intelligent and knowledgeable, yet seemed to be pursuing policies that contradicted long held objectives. Is it that they didn't understand their own policies or did they face constraints that narrow economics did not reveal? Should I conclude that whoever advised them on policy either didn't know as much economics as I or knew a lot of things I didn't know? Of course, the two options were not mutually exclusive.

The first case arose during a discussion of the drug benefits provided to factory workers and their dependents under a particular union contract. I was struck by the fact that the drug benefit did not include some drugs that were rarely prescribed, but which were very costly when they were needed, while providing coverage for some frequently used but inexpensive over-the-counter pharmaceuticals. This arrangement seemed odd: it violated principles of insurance that call for coverage of expensive but rare events, for example, the heart bypass surgery but not the semi-annual blood pressure check-up, and offered little financial protection against the high expenses that surely must have been of concern to union members and their leadership.

When I expressed astonishment about the benefit structure, I was told that this set of benefit choices was the consequence of "union democracy," something that union leadership believed in. I was given a description of the nature of union elections and was reminded that those who run for elective office including union offices as well as government positions find it advantageous and perhaps necessary to remind voters of the benefits that the candidate has delivered or will bring to the electorate. Candidates search for benefits that as many voters as possible have used and that all voters understand and believe they might use. They would prefer to bring home the bacon to all, rather than the filet mignon to some. Of course, the knowledge that one is protected against an unusually high—albeit, unlikely—expenditure is a real benefit; it is—or should be—the reason that so many of us buy insurance. Nevertheless, it is one thing to convince individuals of that kind of a benefit if they have not utilized the care provided—"remember even if you didn't need the medication, some of your brothers did"—as contrasted with the benefit that everyone shared in –"in our last contract we were able to add a drug benefit that helped you, your family, and each and every brother in this union hall." Abstraction is likely to be trumped by experience.

The lesson, of course, is not that economics is wrong and economists mistaken. Nor is it that union leaders behave in an irrational manner and that union democracy—or, since the "problem" is not unique to unions, all democracy—is a "bad" thing. Perhaps a lesson is that all of us have to spend more time educating ourselves and others that "a bird in hand is not always worth two in the bush," that insurance that provides financial protection against life altering expenditures has great value, and that when it has not been necessary to use it one hasn't "wasted one's money." Perhaps the overriding lesson is that we need to invest more resources in voter education. That, however, is for the future. The immediate lesson that I drew was that economic analysis that is bereft of an understanding of the ways that decisions are reached and of context may not be very helpful in understanding human behavior and human arrangements. It was important to understand—as I suspect every political leader would and many college professors wouldn't—that the union contract that appeared to be foolish derived from an understanding of political behavior and principles of political science and sociology, not from ignorance and bad economics. The policy decision that economists and others might have supported would not have passed the test of the next election.

The second incident also relates to arrangements for health insurance and, again, tells of what some would consider non-economic factors that enter into dynamic policy decisions. As most of us are aware and as all of us should be, under existing personal income tax arrangements marginal tax rates increase as taxable income rises—under present law up to a maximum tax rate of 35 percent. As a consequence, an itemized deduction saves an individual in an upper-income bracket more dollars in taxes than the same itemized deduction saves persons with less income and who, therefore, are in a lower tax bracket. The wealthy person who gives $100 to the United Way saves $35 in taxes and, thus, the donation effectively only costs her or him $65; the individual of more modest means who is in the 15 percent tax bracket finds that the government "subsidizes" that gift with $15 and that the charitable deduction costs $85. Such individuals may feel good that the $100 gift only cost $85. Their joy, however, may be tempered by the knowledge that, in what they may consider a perverse manner, the same gift costs their higher income neighbor only $65.

The same phenomenon is found with a certain class of employer-provided benefits of real value which because of legislative decisions reflected in the income tax code are not counted as taxable income to the individual. Thus, for example, since employer provided health insurance is not considered taxable income to the employee—although it is considered a "cost of doing business" for the employer—the fact that it is a non-taxable benefit is of greater "value" to those of higher income, that is, they save more dollars because the benefit is not taxable. The amount of such forgone taxes is considerable: in the fiscal 2009 budget submitted by President Bush the "tax expenditure" associated with non-taxable health insurance was estimated at $168 billion, a figure close to 80 percent of the projected Medicaid budget. One might and should ask whether this is the most appropriate way to "spend"—tax income foregone can be considered the equivalent of an expenditure—almost $200 billion on health care. The answer, of course, may well be "no," but political reality must recognize that, like many deductions and expenditures economists would question, this tax benefit is institutionalized and something that those who have employer provided benefits count on. Since this benefit is worth more to the higher paid employee—I derive a larger benefit than does my secretary—one might expect that the labor movement would favor a different arrangement in which the amount of money the federal purse loses was disbursed in a more equitable manner. That could be accomplished by using tax credits rather than deductions and by providing greater benefits to low and middle income individuals. I had occasion to raise this question with an official of the AFL-CIO. I wondered why the labor movement was willing to live with the existing inequitable arrangement.

I discovered that I did not have to elaborate about the inequity associated with the provision of a greater subsidy to persons who had higher income. He understood the matter fully and quickly made it clear that he was aware of and unhappy with the situation. He explained that labor movement leaders faced a difficult political problem: they feared that raising the issue as a matter to be addressed by the Congress would not guarantee that it would be addressed nor could they be certain that, if addressed, that the final outcome would be more to labor's advantage—legislation changes as it wends its way through the legislative process. Yet, there were costs associated with raising the issue. If it were raised but not dealt with—let alone dealt with in a disadvantageous manner—the labor movement would have taken a position that might come back to haunt it in the next collective bargaining sessions. Management might argue that rather than engaging in inequitable behavior, labor should accept a taxable wage increase in lieu of non-taxable health benefits. The now smaller *after tax* income would not purchase the same level of health insurance benefits than those previously provided (and would become even less over time as health care costs and health insurance premiums rose more rapidly than wages). Thus, as a matter of strategy, labor simply did not want to take a chance on congressional action. The problem was not with labor's failure to understand economics, but with labor's recognition of the vagaries of the political process. To think that all behavior can be understood and explained in economic terms was incorrect. Once again, there was a political dimension to the debate.

This incident underlines the importance of non-economic considerations (even if one might argue that collective bargaining does fall in the economist's domain). It also serves as a reminder that our political process is complex and unpredictable. That has extraordinarily important implications for decision makers and their policy advisers and serves to introduce the third incident, one in which a proposal's uncertain future affects today's decisions. It points up how an unpredictable political environment can affect support for and the possible outcome of proposed legislation. In doing so it reminds us that the policy adviser must be attuned to considerations that often fall outside his or her disciplinary base.

Few of us may remember and it may be difficult to imagine, that when the Clinton universal health insurance program was proposed, the polls showed a high level of support among the general public. Americans felt positively about the initiative and the groundswell of support led many to overlook various problems the legislation would face including its complexity and issues of timing related to the need for enactment of an economic stimulus package, as well as the power of legislators like Representative Dan Rostenkowski, chairman of the House Ways and Means Committee through which the legislation would have to move and Senator Pat Moynihan, long time advocate of speedy action on welfare reform, and their relationships with the president and the first lady. It was virtually taken for granted that the Clinton program or a variant thereof, but nonetheless one that would move the nation a long way toward universal coverage would be enacted.

As a consequence, various large employers who provided health insurance benefits to their employees and insurance carriers whose activities would be materially affected and who were parties of interest tried to study the plan, assess its implications, and monitor changes that might develop as the proposal moved through the congressional legislative process. So it was that two colleagues and I were invited to Detroit by Michigan Blue Cross-Blue Shield, the dominant organization in the state health insurance market, to meet with representatives of one of the big three motor company, one of Michigan's important non-auto manufacturers, and one of the largest public employees unions. We were to discuss an appropriate agenda for research on and modeling of the evolving Clinton plan and ways that we might contribute to efforts at simulating the impact of the legislation as it evolved.

As it happened, I had awakened very early, had turned on the TV in my hotel room and, for the first time, had watched what came to be known as the Harry and Louise commercial. I felt that the ad was extremely powerful and believed it would be very effective. Since others in the meeting had not yet had an opportunity to see Louise and Harry at the kitchen table or hear Louise tell Harry and millions of Americans that she didn't understand the plan and that there must be a simpler way, my concern and skepticism about enactment of the proposed plan was easily dismissed. Our conversation about needed research continued.

Among the various important elements in the Clinton proposal was one that offered massive financial relief to firms that provided health insurance benefits to their retirees. These costs—which had a negative impact on price competition between firms and which were a severe burden on firms in declining industries—would be shifted to the federal government. Such a provision had vast favorable implications for the automobile firm in the room and, as well, for its two old-line American competitors. As we have come to know, as the automotive settlements between the big three and the United Automobile Workers (UAW) in 2007 demonstrate, and as the loan provisions involving the U.S. Treasury and American automobile manufacturers in 2008 document, this very considerable financial burden adversely and significantly affected the competitive pricing position of the big three as contrasted with the foreign auto firms located in the United States who, because of their comparative "youth," had and have many fewer retirees.

Nevertheless, the automobile manufacturing representative seemed to offer no more than tepid support for the Clinton proposal. Finally, with some frustration, if not exasperation, one of my colleagues turned to the auto executive and asked why, given how much the retiree proposal would mean to his company he was so lukewarm and even unenthusiastic about the Clinton program. I had long held the view that given the financial problems of General Motors, Ford, and Chrysler as a direct consequence of their provision of health benefits to their work force and retirees, the only way that one could explain their failure to lobby for national health insurance over all the many years of political debate was as "the triumph of ideology over self interest." Odd as it may have seemed, these firms were negating the lessons that they presumably had learned from Adam Smith. Even so, their failure to support the Clinton program and the billions of dollars they stood to gain seemed to involve more than that.

My colleague did not have to wait long for the auto executive to provide an answer to the question. He explained that the proposal was viewed as a "bribe" designed to garner support. That, however, was not the issue. After all, what some might consider a "bribe" could readily be defined as "enlightened public policy" designed to create a level playing field. Rather, the problem was that his firm believed that the amount involved was so large and its fiscal implications so great that the provision and the relief it would provide would not survive through the legislative process. The final legislation that would emerge was unpredictable, but he believed one thing was certain: whatever was enacted would not contain the favorable aspects that the questioner presumed.

Inevitably, the subsequent problem would be that his firm and the other manufacturers who would join would lose the part of the program from which they would derive extraordinary benefit and be "stuck with" other, perhaps, unfavorable, aspects of the Clinton program from which they would find it difficult, if not impossible, to disengage. They would discover they were trapped into support or forced into a disclaimer that would reveal their narrowness of purpose, i.e., that they didn't care about principles like universality, but only about how much money they might garner. Better to disengage now than engage in what, given the American political system, would inevitably be a very fluid process. What seemed so clear to my colleague and to me—that the firm would be impelled by its economic self interest—was not at all clear when the politics of the situation were factored in.

Once again, the problem was not "economics" but "political economy," that is the application of economics in the unpredictable political world. What would make sense in the abstract world of theory and in the classroom was not applicable in the non-parliamentary system with many loci of power and with little party discipline, a system in which even presidents cannot deliver requisite votes to enact their proposals. That, of course, does not mean that the classroom exercise is irrelevant. It is part, a necessary part, of the economist's education. Furthermore, it is sufficient for those who want to devote their full attention to exercises in pure theory, which are important activities in advancing the discipline of economics. At the same time, it is woefully incomplete for those who want to leave the classroom and apply their theory in a world in which behavior and events are heavily influenced and impelled by variables not classified as economic. Once again we are reminded that economics is useful and powerful but that it is only one of many perspectives and disciplines necessary to fashion policy.

Keep It Simple

In the mid-1960s, I served on a committee established by the Carnegie Corporation to develop programs designed to increase access to health care. Our focus was delivery system change rather than the "usual" agenda encompassing the availability and financing of health insurance and the achievement of universality. Many of the committee members were distinguished physicians who had years of experience in providing medical care, teaching and training students and residents, and conducting research. All of the members were individuals concerned with the distribution of medical care and with the need to make high quality care available to all Americans.

One of the areas of inquiry we focused on dealt with the availability of medical care to rural populations. The Hospital Survey and Construction Act, better known as the Hill-Burton Act, a Truman administration initiative that had been enacted in 1946, was having positive impact on rural health care facility and hospital construction and renovation. In turn, the growth in the number of rural hospitals helped increase the supply of physicians practicing in smaller and less urban communities. Nevertheless, change in the location of physicians and in the practice of medicine came slowly. When, in 1954-1955, I interviewed all North Carolina general practitioners who had opened a practice in the previous three years, few if any of them mentioned "the hospital"—or even whether there was one in their community—as playing a significant role in their choice of a place to practice. Conversely, when these same physicians were interviewed twenty-five years later and their satisfactions and dissatisfactions over the previous two and a half decades of practice were discussed, "the hospital" played a central role in their "story." In the mid-1960s the physicians who practiced in rural areas were overworked and felt lonely and isolated.

The members of the Carnegie committee were well aware of the growth in the number of hospitals, of the increase in availability of care in smaller and rural communities, and of the expansion of miles of paved roads—as a governor of North Carolina claimed to potential voters, "we paved the roads so that you can get to church on Sunday and to the hospital when you're sick." However, the physician members of the committee most of whom were associated with teaching hospitals and university health centers were also aware of the wide disparity between the care—especially, specialty care—available in those teaching centers and the care available in rural communities at some distance from the medical school and university setting. They were cognizant of the fact that one couldn't place a teaching hospital with all its ancillary equipment and appropriate personnel in every town and hamlet in

America, but they were equally cognizant that one didn't respond to the need for care with a statement that "the folks who live there chose to live there."

"Market" aficionados might say, "Free to choose and free to move." Most of us around the Carnegie table felt that statement would be somewhat akin to the suggestion that we do not need mine safety regulations since economic theory suggested that, absent safety regulations, miners would be compensated for the higher risk of accidents by higher wages. We had a problem accepting the view that miners were free not to work in the mine and nevertheless chose to do so. Similarly, the committee did not view rural folk as "losers" who had chosen not to move to urban communities and "having made their beds should now lie in them." Rather, the committee set about trying to think how, within the limits of available resources, one could bring higher quality care to outlying populations.

Eugene Stead, one of the leaders in American medicine and a critical figure in medical education at Duke, felt that the answer lay in "linking" physicians in the smaller and distant communities with physicians in the teaching medical center and thus enabling the primary care physician to discuss the individual patient with the specialist and sub-specialist. The "distant" primary care physician and the specialist teaching hospital physician would communicate, the abilities and power of the medical center would be extended, and as a consequence the quality of care would be raised for the benefit of the patient. All of us were aware that such an arrangement would require negotiation around fee structures and some way of engendering trust that the medical center would not "steal" the patient, but those and similar problems that we could foresee would arise were not the first order of business. Instead, what Gene Stead wanted to do first was to discuss the technology that would make it possible to establish the necessary operating linkage. In order to stimulate that discussion he suggested we invite engineers from Western Electric/Bell Labs, the world-renowned research facility of the Bell telephone system, to one of our meetings. All of us endorsed the idea: the technological imperative led us to believe that the answer must lie in some new technology.

We met and Dr. Stead defined what he saw as the issue: "What do you have on the drawing boards that would yield a more precise diagnosis of the patient's condition by enabling better 'communication' between the physician who was examining a patient and the physician in the established medical center many miles distant." The engineers were equally clear: "That's not how we approach a problem. We'll ask you in quite specific terms what information you might need to improve care, tell you what technologies we have that might enable the necessary information transfer, tell you something about the cost of transfer, and thereby encourage you to consider alternatives as well as whether the presumed needs you have defined are true "needs" or "conveniences." They began their inquiry. "Is it necessary for the physician at the university medical center, say Duke, to be able to see the patient in the other doctor's office?" When the answer was "yes" they asked whether that meant in a continuous manner (as say, on television) or in a snapshot manner, say a still picture transmitted every six or eight seconds. Gene responded that continuous pictures were preferable. The engineers responded that, of course, that technology could be provided, but that they had raised the alternative option because the additional telephone transmission lines required for the transmission of continuous images would add quite substantially to costs.

Dr. Stead decided that periodic snapshot pictures would suffice, that the benefits of a continuous display were not that large and were not likely to be worth the additional cost. "What about color? Would you like the pictures to be in color or would black and white suffice?" The physicians around the table agreed that there were occasions when color could aid in diagnosis and would be useful. Again the reply was that color could be made available, but only at significant additional cost. Again the response was that given the additional costs of color, black and white transmission could and would suffice. And so it went: the engineers inquired about smell and indicated that technologies existed that would permit the Duke physician to smell the distant patient. Again that seemed "necessary" till it became clear that, too, would be quite costly. The number of times that the distant physician could not describe smells accurately or at least adequately, the number of times that the diagnosis would be different if the Duke physician could smell the patient was too low to justify the added expenditure. What turned out to be the final interchange took place around "feel." The engineers explained that they could put sensors on each of the fingers of each of the two physicians who were communicating and that as the one physician palpated the patient, the sensations he or she felt would be transmitted to the second physician. Though this seemed advantageous, Dr. Stead ended up rejecting the technology. The reason, of course, was the high cost associated with the transmission of the sensations across the multiple telephone lines.

But there was a second reason as well. After a pause, Gene Stead turned to the engineers and to the committee and quite dramatically announced that he had come to realize that the requisite technology to enable the appropriate and necessary communication already existed. He confessed that he had asked the wrong question and had misled everyone when he inquired "what's on the drawing board." In fact, he already had a working model of the requisite technology on his night table at home. It was a black mechanism with a roughly five-inch by nine-inch footprint. The instrument was called a telephone. That technology enabled his residents in the hospital to reach their mentor and communicate with him when he was at home. The critical thing was that the resident knew that when he or she called, someone would answer. The absence of advanced technology wasn't the bottleneck that prevented a relationship between the physicians at Duke and the physicians in distant parts of North Carolina. Rather, the bottleneck was that no one had set up a system that linked these physicians and that assured that when the one called, a responsible individual would be at the other end of the line.

The session with the Bell Labs engineers had proven immensely useful. It had enabled us to see that the problem we were addressing was not one of "technology," but of "system." Of course there are places and times where changes in technology provide a breakthrough in the way work can be carried on effectively. Yet, a focus on technology may keep one from examining the organization of the "system," such questions as who performs which tasks or how information flows, is processed, and exchanged. Technological "solutions" are appealing: dollars are being set aside, hardware is being purchased or software installed, something is being done. There is a sense of activity, things are not standing still, and latest advances are being incorporated. Furthermore, installation of new technology permits one to claim that the organization is "on top of things," is cutting edge, and is incorporating the very latest research products. Conversely, altering systems seems a bit prosaic and, once explained, somewhat self-evident. Observers may question why such presumably inexpensive and obvious changes weren't made earlier. Surely, twenty sensors on twenty fingers is a more exciting and dramatic "advance" than relying on the telephone, assigning new responsibilities, and reorganizing tasks. And drama is useful: it motivates people and leads to participation, at least until the drama wears off.

But complex and costly answers are not necessary if simpler answers will suffice. The principle of Occam's razor, the principle of parsimony, "What can be done with fewer [assumptions] is done in vain with more" remains alive. It is worth testing the telephone hypothesis and designing the human systems to enable the phone to be used effectively before investing in live color television pictures, a sense of smell, and touch and discovering that the additional complexity added little since, unless the human systems are redesigned, the new technology would not work effectively.

The issue of simplicity and complexity extends far beyond the use of technology, although, it should be clear that the very presence of new technology often leads policy makers and analysts to favor the adoption of complex approaches and to negate consideration of simpler ones. After all, there are firms that produce and sales personnel that sell the new technology while system change though less costly is a process internal to the organization. Nevertheless while there is a certain appeal inherent in high end technology, there is a certain advantage in older technologies. Consider the modern cell phone that can do so many things that a number of firms now market a "simple" phone that is more easily used. We have all been in homes which have a VCR, DVD, coffee maker, micro-wave oven, and other electric appliance whose clocks are blinking because no one is quite certain how to reset the correct time after a power outage? I once was told how fortunate the nation was that by 1965 computer capability had increased sufficiently to enable the design of Medicare to incorporate deductibles and co-insurance: "Imagine how difficult, if not impossible, it would have been to track the deductible if we didn't have the requisite computer capability. We might not have been able to have Medicare!" Of course, the appropriate response is to note that we might have had a different Medicare, one without the deductible. The presence of the computer enabled us to structure Medicare in a particular, but not necessarily better, way.

Simplicity has other virtues. Consider the various proposed designs for universal health insurance. Many of them call for "mandates" entailing numerous steps involving initial enrollment, the periodic determination of income and level of assistance, the approval of insurance benefit packages, the opportunity for change in enrollment, the nature of employer involvement and financial underwriting, the administration of retroactive penalties for failure to enroll, and so forth. Each step introduces another opportunity for "error" and those various errors are additive and cumulative. It would be easy to take pride in a high level of performance at each step in the process and yet end up with a program that badly missed the mark of universality. It is not enough to be able to claim great efficiency in the performance of tasks that are inherently in-efficient, that is, tasks that would be unnecessary under a simpler and more efficient design.

It is indeed true that sometimes the problem at hand cannot be solved through a "simple" change and a "simple" approach or if solved in that manner might conflict with other values. That is the nature of part of the debate around Medicare for All, or what is often called a "single-payer" approach, as the way to reach univer-sal health insurance and as contrasted with employer, individual and family mandates or tax-credit "solutions." The latter are more complex and bureaucratic and in that sense less efficient, but are nonetheless viewed by many as preferable because they involve less "government" And some place a high value on that character-istic. Nevertheless, in such debates it is worth remembering Gene Stead's telephone. Sometimes—though not always—the answer is quite close at hand. Sometimes—though not always—the failure to consider "simpler" approaches leads to such program characteristics as are found in Part D Medicare: the unfortunate "donut holes," the annual private sector changes in premiums, formularies, and therefore enrollment choices, and the confusion inherent in the design characteristics. The issue can be put succinctly: "If the program looks like a Rube Goldberg creation, put it in a cartoon not in the legislative hopper." In formulating policy there is no premium for unnecessary complexity.

Epilogue

Some readers might wonder which of the various policy lessons or stories I have recounted is my favorite. That seems to me to be a reasonable kind of question and one that I have asked myself. Of course, the answer is heavily dependent on what one means by "favorite." Which of the many possible criteria is to be given the greatest weight: the lesson that most readily can be applied; the one that deals with broad issues of citizenship and that transcends issues involved in policy advising; the story that best warns against specific mistakes; the event that had the largest continuing impact on me? Surely, the favorite ought to be one that illustrates what I would consider the most significant point and the one most likely to be overlooked.

Nevertheless, though reasonable, the question is not very important. The reader who has read the book may want to guess my preference to satisfy his or her curiosity, but I rather suspect that the guess will be determined by a mixture of what the reader relates to as well as what he or she imagines I might prefer. The first – the reader's preference – is of much greater significance.

But before any reader considers the matter, there is one more lesson and story that merits – indeed, requires – telling. After all it is possible that some who have read the text and have found it interesting and even relevant to the ways to think about policy, nevertheless believe the lessons do not apply to them. These readers may stand aloof because they do not believe they have the kinds of jobs or involvements that provide the opportunity to influence policy decisions, or at least decisions that would "make a difference." What can one individual – unless he or she is the president or an important legislator, judge, or executive – accomplish? True, within the family and perhaps the enterprise with which that individual is associated (if it is sufficiently small) one person's views and efforts may have an impact. Yet, on the "affairs of state," on issues of government policy on such matters as taxes, expenditures, domestic and foreign affairs, on the things that are of prime importance in setting the context for our private behaviors what difference can one "small" individual make?

The reader who takes that attitude and is tempted to remove him or her self from the action would perhaps be better able to resist that temptation by learning from the recounting of the remaining story. It may not become the reader's favorite anecdote, but the lesson I believe it teaches is relevant to all the other policy matters I have raised.

One Person Can Make a Difference

All of us who follow sports are aware that in some games one play or one player can make all the difference. We recognize the remarkable catch, the unfortunate fumble, the home run, the error, the half-court three point shot, the various plays that are so exceptional that even in a team sport the outcome may be dependent on that one player. So it also is in the arts. Each contributor is different as is each contribution: Mahler is not Mozart, Shaw is not Shakespeare and Picasso is not Pissarro, though each and all of them were exceptional.

At the same time, most of us do not really believe that, except perhaps in a small committee, our single vote will make a difference, that our letter to the editor or op-ed piece will have a substantial impact in the marketplace of ideas and influence events, or that our latest research finding – at least in the social sciences – will have a dramatic immediate impact on the human condition. Yet, many of us do vote, write letters, and contribute op-ed pieces. And many of us do our research believing that even if ours is only one study it will not stand alone and that when added to all the other studies it will, over time, enhance and influence our and our colleagues' understanding. We behave as if those actions are the membership dues we feel obliged to pay in order to belong to the club called "society."

Nevertheless, on one occasion I believed and tried to convince a close friend and colleague that it was time to go home: "Come on; let's quit. Your efforts won't make any difference." It happened on a late Friday afternoon in the spring of 1963 when I was a staff member at the Council of Economic Advisers. It was a bit after six in the early evening and having cleared off my desk I was ready to go home. It was only a few short blocks to the corner where there was a stop for a bus that went up Connecticut Avenue. Though "local" buses ran quite frequently, there was a real incentive to get out by 6:20 and catch the last bus that operated on an express schedule and made its first stop some miles away at Porter Street and its next one well beyond, at Chevy Chase Circle. I would get off at Porter and my close friend and fellow council staff member, Bob Lampman, would get off at Chevy Chase Circle. Catching the express enabled me to save a lot of time and Bob saved even more.

So on that Friday, a little after six, I went into Lampman's spacious office. I reminded him that it was time to leave and urged him to do so for there was little time to spare if he and I were to catch the last express bus. Bob told me that he couldn't leave. The latest data on the distribution of income – his field of interest and his professional area of expertise and responsibility at the Council – had been released that day. He wanted to stay and write a memo on the implication of the new figures and place it in Chairman Heller's "in box." Even with all my "dedication" to helping to get America moving again, I argued with Bob. I reminded him that we could be quite certain that Heller's in box was full since Walter seldom turned to it to read the various memos in it. Important matters were raised orally and his excellent executive secretary personally handed him any memoranda that needed action. Most memoranda were buried in the in box, though occasionally they were exhumed and, if still relevant, were dealt with. I argued that, given the backlog, at best it would be a long time before Lampman's latest memo would be read. Bob could certainly write the memorandum on Monday and it would most probably be read at the same time than if he wrote it this Friday night. Nothing would be lost if he went home; it made no difference. Bob insisted that he'd stay. It was part of his "job" and the right thing to do. Certainly the memo could wait; certainly the memo shouldn't wait. I left by myself, impressed and, perhaps, even a bit puzzled, by Bob's commitment.

When I came in on Monday, I was chastened to find that on my desk there was a memorandum that had been dictated by Heller over the weekend. Walter had come in on Saturday morning and decided to catch up on things by starting at the top of the in box and working his way down through it as far as he was able. There, at the very top, was Lampman's discussion of the latest data on America's income distribution and their implications. Walter's memo asked Bob to be the lead person on thinking through what the administration might do to reduce existing income disparities and what economic policies it might favor to deal with the problems faced by those at the bottom of the distribution, by the impact of those disparities. I was to help Bob think through the potential attributes of an anti-poverty program.

To say that is where "The War on Poverty" began would be an exaggeration. Policies are not adopted simply because one person writes a convincing memo; the road to a war on poverty required many steps. Indeed, Heller was already considering what progressive policies might follow the tax cut that had been proposed – but not yet enacted – to help reduce unemployment. He had not yet turned to the development of a comprehensive program to fight poverty, but had begun to refer to the need to deal with problems of the poor in various "trial balloon" speeches he delivered in the spring of 1963. Yet, I am prepared to argue that the Lampman memo, though not a sufficient condition, was a necessary one for the development of a comprehensive program that attempted to deal with existing income inequalities. It moved what had been and what might have remained a few sentences and paragraphs in speeches to the agenda of active consideration. It provided the occasion for Walter to raise the issue of poverty and income distribution with a memorandum to the president.

Importantly, the memorandum might have had little impact had Bob decided to yield to my entreaties to join me on the express bus. We do not know when the memo would have been read had it not been available that Saturday and, whether at some later time and under different conditions it would have been accorded the same priority. Timing may not be everything – some of us, after all, remember when we were told "it's all about location, location,

location…" – but certainly it is important. But timing is not entirely fortuitous. Bob Lampman didn't just happen to review the most recent income distribution data on that given Friday because the thought struck him to do so or because he had nothing better to do. And having reviewed the various statistics he didn't just decide to inform the Council members of the data and of their implication. He wrote his memorandum that very evening because he knew that he should do so, because it was his responsibility. It is, therefore, no accident that many years later the former Council member, Jim Tobin, by then a Nobel economist, described Bob as "the intellectual architect of the War on Poverty."[1] Without him, we might have had a skirmish, but most assuredly not more. The title that Dean Acheson had chosen to describe his years at the State Department, *Present at the Creation*, could have described Bob Lampman and the War on Poverty. And it began with a Friday evening memo.

I do believe there is "a tide in the affairs of men." Even so, I also believe one person can make a difference. Bob Lampman did so and many other Bob Lampmans have done so. There is a lesson in this for all of us and that lesson does not apply solely to the great affairs of state and public policy. It applies as well, though in far less dramatic fashion, to all of us in everyday life. Fortunate the person who can feel he or she made a real difference be that person the plumber who diagnosed and fixed the leak, the teacher who sparked a child, the artist whose creation was unique and could not have been done by someone else, the civil servant who wrote the memorandum. One thing we know about that person and that difference: it would not have happened had there not been the effort and the attempt.

And there is one thing more. As the individual may make a difference by his or her actions, so too those various actions make a difference on the individual. After the assassination of President Kennedy I watched television and saw the long lines – over 100,000 persons – shuffling through the rotunda of the Capital when the bier was there before the burial in Arlington National Cemetery. A neighbor stopped by our house. Before leaving he asked how it was that I, who had worked for the president, was not in that mile long line and I responded that after all I could see so much more on television. I have regretted that since that day for I have come to understand that there are events – Selma and the March on Washington quickly come to mind, but there are many more – that call upon one to be a participant, not a spectator. The student/activist who decides to work on a campaign for a candidate or for a cause will recall it for years to come and will draw sustenance from it. The memo, written that Friday eve, about the distribution of income made a difference in helping set an agenda. It most certainly meant that when President Johnson took the reins of office, there already was a set of ideas to place before him. That set of ideas impelled him to declare a War on Poverty. But I rather think, and have reason to believe I am correct, that the fact that Bob wrote the memo and, as a consequence, the many discussion papers that followed, also had a positive impact on him. They surely had an impact on me and, perhaps, through me on you, the reader.

This manuscript was being edited when Senator Edward Kennedy dies. Some of the most important lessons in this book were learned in my interactions with the senior senator from Massachusetts. Ultimately the words I have written in an effort to improve the public policy process are based on a fundamental belief that government can work and that it can make a positive difference in our lives. Edward Kennedy's life of public service provides ample evidence of the validity of that belief.

Notes

Introduction

1. A brief version of this story is found in Isaac M. Fein, *The Making of an American Jewish Community: The History of Baltimore Jewry from 1773 to 1920* (Philadelphia, PA: Jewish Publication Society of America, 1971), pp. vii-viii.
2. Molière in *Le Bourgeois Gentilehomme*, act 2, sc. 4, as quoted in Fred R. Shapiro, ed., *The Yale Book of Quotations* (New Haven, CT: Yale University Press, 2006), p. 530, Molière 7.
3. Edward H. Carr, *What is History?* (New York: Alfred A. Knopf, 1962), pp. 26, 54.

Chapter 1

1. Rashi Fein, *The Economics of Mental Illness* (New York: Basic Books Inc., 1958).
2. Michael Jonas, *Boston Globe* (August 5, 2007), p. D1.

Chapter 2

1. Rashi Fein, "What Is Wrong With the Language of Medicine?" *New England Journal of Medicine*, 306; No. 14 (April 8, 1982), pp. 863-864.
2. Edward R. Murrow, on his Columbia LP recording entitled "I Can Hear It Now" (and possibly elsewhere). The full quotation occurs in Murrow's introduction to his Churchill war speech excerpts, as Churchill takes office in 1940: "Now the hour had come for him to mobilize the English language, and send it into battle, a spearhead of hope for Britain and the world."
3. Fred R. Shapiro, *op. cit.*, "Campañia General de Tabacos de Filipinas v. Collector of Internal Revenue (dissenting opinion) (1927)," p. 368, Holmes 36.
4. As cited in Simon James, *Dictionary of Economic Quotations*, Second Edition, Reprinted as a Helix Book (Totowa, NJ: Rowman and Allanheld 1984), Number 41 (Speech, 1936), p. 177.

5.   Fred R. Shapiro, *op. cit.,* "Yale Towne v. Eisner" (1918), p. 367, Holmes.
6.   Marjorie Hunter, *New York Times*, October 17, 1961, p. 45.
7.   Jonathan Randal, *New York Times*, November 24, 1967, p. 28.
8.   From "The Words and Music of World War II," 1991 and 2001 Columbia Legacy C2K 48516. CD2 Track 1.
9.   Brian Abel Smith and Kay Titmuss, eds. in *Social Policy: An Introduction* (London: George Allen and Unwin, Limited, 1974 and U.S. Pantheon Books, A Division of Random House, New York, 1975), pp. 150-151. The essay is a postscript to the posthumous collection of lectures by Richard Titmuss.

Chapter 3

1.   *Economic Report of the President Transmitted to the Congress January 1962 Together with the Annual Report of the Council of Economic Advisers* (Washington, DC: United States Government Printing Office, 1962), pp.108-143 and especially pp. 117-123.
2.   Theodore Sorenson, *Counselor: A Life at the Edge of History* (New York: HarperCollins, 2008), p. 209.
3.   Theodore Sorenson, *Kennedy* (New York, Harper & Row Publishers, 1965), pp. 362-353.
4.   Rashi Fein, *The Doctor Shortage: An Economic Diagnosis* (Washington, DC: The Brookings Institution, 1967).
5.   Rashi Fein, "On Measuring Economic Benefits of Health Programs" (pp. 181-220) in Gordon McLaughlin, ed. *Medical History and Medical Care: A Symposium of Perspectives* (London: Oxford University Press, 1971).
6.   Oliver Wendell Holmes, Jr. "In Our Youth Our Hearts Were Touched With Fire," Memorial Day Address, May 30, 1884 in Keene, NH, found at people.virginia.edu/~mmd5f/memorial.htm.
7.   Many sources attribute this to David Lloyd George, but cite no particular address or source. Similar quotations are attributed to other individuals and are found in other cultures.

Chapter 4

1.   Douglas MacKinnon, *New York Times,* May 21, 2002, p. A21.

Epilogue

1.   Tobin on Lampman As cited in "A Commemorative History of the Institute for Research on Poverty, 1966-2006," http://www.irp.wisc.edu/newsevents/other/appam-irp40/irphistory.htm.

Index

budget,
    crisis, 36, 167
    debates, 33
    issues, 120
    process, 94-95
    program budgeting, 21-23
    working with budgets, 50-51
Bureau of Labor Statistics, 51
Bureau of the Budget, 6, 72, 151

Carr, Edward, 10-11
Carter, Jimmy, 104, 145-146
civil rights, 38-39, 75, 81, 90, 101, 125
Clinton, Bill, 150, 173-176
Cohen, Wilbur, 84
Comprehensive Health Insurance Program (CHIP), 107
Coombs, Philip, 45
Council of Economic Advisers (CEA), 3-4, 6, 39-40, 42-44, 65-66, 69, 72, 83-86, 90, 151, 187

Department of Health, Education, and Welfare (HEW), 21-23, 84, 90, 151

economics,
    as a discipline, 7-8
    constrained view, 15
    debates, 28-30
    elasticity of demand, 50-51
    Gross National Product (GNP), 18-20
    Increasing U.S. growth, 67-82
    relation to medicine, 17-18, 21, 55, 84-88, 134, 152
    theory, 17
Economics of Mental Illness, The, 15, 18
economists,
    analytical framework, 93
    as social policy advisers, 30-33, 44, 49, 53, 56, 91-92, 143-151
    considerations, 89

education and training, 4, 7-8, 16-17, 20, 88, 168, 176
    roles and responsibilities, 138-140, 169-173
    social medicine, 64
    talking "economics," 65-66
    teaching, 14, 45
    use of mathematics, 8-9, 16, 168
Eisenhower, Dwight D., 102

George, David Lloyd, 103
Gordon, Kermit, 72-76, 85-87

Harvard Medical School, 31, 54, 57, 90-95, 119-123, 142, 256
health policy, 88, 106, 137
Heller, Walter, 28, 40-41, 43, 69, 72, 87, 187-188
Holmes, Oliver Wendell, Jr., 35, 96

Johnson, Lyndon Baines, 11, 21, 23, 72, 74-77, 80, 90-91, 104-105, 111, 190

Kefauver, Estes, 84-88
Kennedy, Edward, 104, 107, 112-114, 121, 145-152
Kennedy, John F., 3-4, 6, 39, 44, 46, 67, 73, 84, 88, 100
King, Mel, 123-125
Knowles, John, 93
Krevans, Julius, 30

legislation,
    changes during legislative process, 172-175
    crafting legislation, 129, 145-146, 150
    health, 81-82, 84, 113-114, 149
    implementing, 103
    importance of names, 29

Machlup, Fritz, 8-9, 18